Neuromuscular Disorders in Children and Adolescents

Neuromuscular Disorders in Children and Adolescents

Editor

Rudolf Korinthenberg

MDPI • Basel • Beijing • Wuhan • Barcelona • Belgrade • Manchester • Tokyo • Cluj • Tianjin

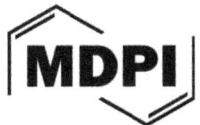

Editor
Rudolf Korinthenberg
Research Ethics Committee
Albert-Ludwigs University
of Freiburg
Freiburg
Germany

Editorial Office
MDPI
St. Alban-Anlage 66
4052 Basel, Switzerland

This is a reprint of articles from the Special Issue published online in the open access journal *Children* (ISSN 2227-9067) (available at: www.mdpi.com/journal/children/special_issues/Neuromuscular_Disorders_Children_Adolescents).

For citation purposes, cite each article independently as indicated on the article page online and as indicated below:

LastName, A.A.; LastName, B.B.; LastName, C.C. Article Title. *Journal Name* **Year**, *Volume Number*, Page Range.

ISBN 978-3-0365-4070-2 (Hbk)
ISBN 978-3-0365-4069-6 (PDF)

© 2022 by the authors. Articles in this book are Open Access and distributed under the Creative Commons Attribution (CC BY) license, which allows users to download, copy and build upon published articles, as long as the author and publisher are properly credited, which ensures maximum dissemination and a wider impact of our publications.

The book as a whole is distributed by MDPI under the terms and conditions of the Creative Commons license CC BY-NC-ND.

Contents

About the Editor vii

Preface to "Neuromuscular Disorders in Children and Adolescents" ix

Rudolf Korinthenberg
Special Issue "Neuromuscular Disorders in Children and Adolescents"
Reprinted from: *Children* **2022**, *9*, 558, doi:10.3390/children9040558 1

Rudolf Korinthenberg, Regina Trollmann, Barbara Plecko, Georg M. Stettner, Markus Blankenburg and Joachim Weis et al.
Differential Diagnosis of Acquired and Hereditary Neuropathies in Children and Adolescents—Consensus-Based Practice Guidelines
Reprinted from: *Children* **2021**, *8*, 687, doi:10.3390/children8080687 5

Agnieszka Cebula, Maciej Cebula and Ilona Kopyta
Muscle Ultrasonographic Elastography in Children: Review of the Current Knowledge and Application
Reprinted from: *Children* **2021**, *8*, 1042, doi:10.3390/children8111042 25

Christina T. Rüsch, Ursula Knirsch, Daniel M. Weber, Marianne Rohrbach, André Eichenberger and Jürg Lütschg et al.
Etiology of Carpal Tunnel Syndrome in a Large Cohort of Children
Reprinted from: *Children* **2021**, *8*, 624, doi:10.3390/children8080624 39

Kyung-Sun Park
Two Approaches for a Genetic Analysis of Pompe Disease: A Literature Review of Patients with Pompe Disease and Analysis Based on Genomic Data from the General Population
Reprinted from: *Children* **2021**, *8*, 601, doi:10.3390/children8070601 49

Katherine D. Mathews, Kristin M. Conway, Amber M. Gedlinske, Nicholas Johnson, Natalie Street and Russell J. Butterfield et al.
Characteristics of Clinical Trial Participants with Duchenne Muscular Dystrophy: Data from the Muscular Dystrophy Surveillance, Tracking, and Research Network (MD STAR*net*)
Reprinted from: *Children* **2021**, *8*, 835, doi:10.3390/children8100835 61

Adela Della Marina, Marc Pawlitzki, Tobias Ruck, Andreas van Baalen, Nadine Vogt and Bernd Schweiger et al.
Clinical Course, Myopathology and Challenge of Therapeutic Intervention in Pediatric Patients with Autoimmune-Mediated Necrotizing Myopathy
Reprinted from: *Children* **2021**, *8*, 721, doi:10.3390/children8090721 73

Minsu Gu and Hyun-Ho Kong
Improvement in Fine Manual Dexterity in Children with Spinal Muscular Atrophy Type 2 after Nusinersen Injection: A Case Series
Reprinted from: *Children* **2021**, *8*, 1039, doi:10.3390/children8111039 85

Meaghann S. Weaver, Alice Yuroff, Sarah Sund, Scott Hetzel and Matthew A. Halanski
Quality of Life Outcomes According to Differential Nusinersen Exposure in Pediatric Spinal Muscular Atrophy
Reprinted from: *Children* **2021**, *8*, 604, doi:10.3390/children8070604 93

Matthew A. Halanski, Rewais Hanna, James Bernatz, Max Twedt, Sarah Sund and Karen Patterson et al.
Sagittal Plane Deformities in Children with SMA2 following Posterior Spinal Instrumentation
Reprinted from: *Children* **2021**, *8*, 703, doi:10.3390/children8080703 . . . . **103**

Akshata Huddar, Kiran Polavarapu, Veeramani Preethish-Kumar, Mainak Bardhan, Gopikrishnan Unnikrishnan and Saraswati Nashi et al.
Expanding the Phenotypic Spectrum of *ECEL1*-Associated Distal Arthrogryposis
Reprinted from: *Children* **2021**, *8*, 909, doi:10.3390/children8100909 . . . . **117**

Hye-Chan Ahn, Do-Hoon Kim, Chul-Hyun Cho, Jun-Chul Byun and Jang-Hyuk Cho
Neuralgic Amyotrophy with Concomitant Hereditary Neuropathy with Liability to Pressure Palsy as a Cause of Dropped Shoulder in a Child after Human Papillomavirus Vaccination: A Case Report
Reprinted from: *Children* **2022**, *9*, 528, doi:10.3390/children9040528 . . . . **129**

About the Editor

Rudolf Korinthenberg

Rudolf Korinthenberg is a Senior German pediatrician and pediatric neurologist. Following his undergraduate studies and residency at Muenster University, Germany, he served as a consultant at Mannheim Clinical Center, University of Heidelberg. From 1990 to 2017, he was the medical director of the division of Neuropediatrics and Muscular Disorders, Center of Pediatrics and Adolescent Medicine, University Hospital of Freiburg University, Germany. He is a member of national and international scientific societies, amongst them the German Muscular Dystrophy Network and the international TREAT-NMD Network and Alliance. He received several awards in the field of neuromuscular diseases. Since his retirement from clinical duties, he holds the position of the chairman of the Research Ethics Committee of Freiburg University, Germany.

Preface to "Neuromuscular Disorders in Children and Adolescents"

The term "neuromuscular disorders" includes acquired and inherited diseases of the peripheral nervous system affecting structures such as the spinal motor neurons and sensory root ganglia, cranial and peripheral nerves with their axons and myelin sheaths, neuromuscular synapses, and muscle fibers. Our call at the beginning of 2021 resulted in 12 peer-reviewed publications covering a wide range of topics in the field of neuromuscular disorders in children and adolescents. This Special Issue contains a collection of these studies and reviews covering the broad field of peripheral nerve and muscle disorders. I would like to thank all the authors who have contributed to the success of this issue.

Rudolf Korinthenberg
Editor

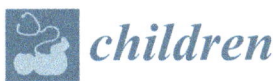

Editorial

Special Issue "Neuromuscular Disorders in Children and Adolescents"

Rudolf Korinthenberg

Research Ethics Committee, University of Freiburg, 79106 Freiburg, Germany; rudolf.korinthenberg@uniklinik-freiburg.de

Citation: Korinthenberg, R. Special Issue "Neuromuscular Disorders in Children and Adolescents". *Children* 2022, 9, 558. https://doi.org/10.3390/children9040558

Received: 14 January 2022
Accepted: 30 March 2022
Published: 14 April 2022

Publisher's Note: MDPI stays neutral with regard to jurisdictional claims in published maps and institutional affiliations.

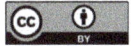

Copyright: © 2022 by the author. Licensee MDPI, Basel, Switzerland. This article is an open access article distributed under the terms and conditions of the Creative Commons Attribution (CC BY) license (https://creativecommons.org/licenses/by/4.0/).

Our call for contributions in early 2021 resulted in 10 peer-reviewed publications by the end of the year covering a wide range of topics in the field of neuromuscular diseases in children and adolescents. The term "neuromuscular disorders" includes acquired and inherited diseases of the peripheral nervous system affecting structures such as the spinal motor neurons and sensory root ganglia, cranial and peripheral nerves with their axons and myelin sheaths, neuromuscular synapses and muscle fibres. The articles in this Special Issue deal with the aetiology, diagnostics and treatment of the resulting diseases.

Rudolf Korinthenberg and colleagues from Germany report on their practice guideline on the differential diagnosis of acquired and hereditary neuropathies in children and adolescents. This guideline is based on a structured consensus process of experts in the field delegated by the participating medical–scientific societies in German-speaking countries. The guideline contains detailed recommendations for the diagnostic work-up of such neuropathies, including the ever-growing field of genetic neuropathies of the Charcot-Marie-Tooth type [1].

Agnieszka Cebula and her colleagues from Poland provide an overview of the current state of knowledge and application of the ultrasound elastography of muscles. This relatively new imaging technique for the qualitative and quantitative assessment of tissue elasticity is already used to examine various organs in adults, but experience in children is still limited. Analysis of the existing literature has been hampered by widely varying protocols in terms of instrument settings and probe positions. However, once the methods have been standardised, the authors expect this non-invasive method to be of great benefit for the diagnosis and follow-up of both natural history and treatment effects in diseases as diverse as muscular dystrophies and cerebral palsy [2].

Christina T. Rüsch and colleagues from Switzerland report on a large cohort of 38 children with carpal tunnel syndrome. Unlike in adults, the aetiology in these children was rarely idiopathic, but mostly secondary to tumours; vascular malformations; and—in these specialised centres—metabolic diseases, such as mucopolysaccharidoses. Electrophysiological examinations and nerve ultrasound were successful in establishing the diagnosis [3].

Kyung-Sun Park from Seoul, Korea, investigated two approaches to genetic analysis of Pompe disease in Korean and Japanese patients and in genome databases of the respective general populations. Approximately 50% of the pathogenic or likely pathogenic variants found in unaffected carriers were also found in affected patients with Pompe disease. The carrier frequency of Pompe disease in Koreans and Japanese patients was estimated to be 1.7% and 0.7%, respectively, and the predicted genetic prevalence was 1:13,657 and 1:78,013, respectively [4].

Katherine D. Mathew and her colleagues from the MD STAR network, USA, report on the characteristics of participants in clinical trials with Duchenne muscular dystrophy (DMD). DMD is the most common and one of the most severe neuromuscular diseases in children and adolescents. New treatment approaches have been under development for several years. For the planning of such clinical trials, it is important to assess the feasibility of the data presented and improve access to participation for those affected [5].

Adela Della Marina and her group from Germany report on the clinical course, myopathology and treatment challenges in two patients with autoimmune-mediated necrotising myopathy. This very rare disease can easily be confused with hereditary muscular dystrophy due to its clinical and pathological features. However, the possibility of immunosuppressive treatment makes correct diagnosis extremely important [6].

Minsu Gu and Hyun-Ho Kong from Korea report an improvement in fine manual dexterity in a small series of five children with spinal muscular atrophy type 2 after 18 months of treatment with nusinersen. While improvement in gross motor function has been repeatedly demonstrated, manual dexterity is also of great importance for daily tasks and quality of life. Such functional tests should be included in routine care and also in further large-scale clinical trials [7].

Meaghann S. Weaver and her colleagues from the USA studied several quality-of-life outcomes in 35 patients with varying severity of paediatric spinal muscular atrophy and their families. They report different positive and negative changes depending on the stage of nusinersen treatment, i.e., at initiation and during long-term treatment. This is important information for all professionals caring for this patient group [8].

Matthew A. Halanski and his co-authors from the USA report on the long-term follow-up of 32 children with SMA2 after posterior spinal instrumentation for progressive scoliosis. Scoliosis is a common orthopaedic complication in the natural history of SMA type 2, and its only effective treatment is surgery. However, secondary deformities may occur in the long term due to subsequent spinal growth. The authors describe postoperative deformities in the sagittal plane and their preconditions and consequences [9].

Akshata Huddar and co-workers from India report on three patients from two families suffering from ECEL1-associated distal arthrogryposis type D. These observations expand the phenotypic spectrum of this already known disorder, including clinical and MRI data. In particular, perinatal complications due to congenital contractures may lead to a misdiagnosis of perinatal damage [10].

Neuromuscular diseases encompass an enormous spectrum of acquired and genetic diseases, from Guillain-Barré syndrome to CMT neuropathy, and from congenital malformations to progressive muscular dystrophies. The correct and timely diagnosis and appropriate treatment are of paramount importance to patients and their families. While much of the treatment still relies on symptomatic measures to improve quality of life, there are new, more effective treatments for some of these diseases [see more on https://treat-nmd.org/resources-support/care-overview/] (accessed on 1 March 2022).

Funding: This research received no external funding.

Conflicts of Interest: The author declares no conflict of interest.

References

1. Korinthenberg, R.; Trollmann, R.; Plecko, B.; Stettner, G.M.; Blankenburg, M.; Weis, J.; Schoser, B.; Müller-Felber, W.; Lochbuehler, N.; Hahn, G.; et al. Differential Diagnosis of Acquired and Hereditary Neuropathies in Children and Adolescents—Consensus-Based Practice Guidelines. *Children* **2021**, *8*, 687. [CrossRef] [PubMed]
2. Cebula, A.; Cebula, M.; Kopyta, I. Muscle Ultrasonographic Elastography in Children: Review of the Current Knowledge and Application. *Children* **2021**, *8*, 1042. [CrossRef] [PubMed]
3. Rüsch, C.T.; Knirsch, U.; Weber, D.M.; Rohrbach, M.; Eichenberger, A.; Lütschg, J.; Weber, K.; Broser, P.J.; Stettner, G.M. Etiology of Carpal Tunnel Syndrome in a Large Cohort of Children. *Children* **2021**, *8*, 624. [CrossRef] [PubMed]
4. Park, K.-S. Two Approaches for a Genetic Analysis of Pompe Disease: A Literature Review of Patients with Pompe Disease and Analysis Based on Genomic Data from the General Population. *Children* **2021**, *8*, 601. [CrossRef] [PubMed]
5. Mathews, K.D.; Conway, K.M.; Gedlinske, A.M.; Johnson, N.; Street, N.; Butterfield, R.J.; Hung, M.; Ciafaloni, E.; Romitti, P.A. Characteristics of Clinical Trial Participants with Duchenne Muscular Dystrophy: Data from the Muscular Dystrophy Surveillance, Tracking, and Research Network (MD STARnet). *Children* **2021**, *8*, 835. [CrossRef] [PubMed]

6. Della Marina, A.; Pawlitzki, M.; Ruck, T.; van Baalen, A.; Vogt, N.; Schweiger, B.; Hertel, S.; Kölbel, H.; Wiendl, H.; Preuße, C.; et al. Clinical Course, Myopathology and Challenge of Therapeutic Intervention in Pediatric Patients with Autoimmune-Mediated Necrotizing Myopathy. *Children* **2021**, *8*, 721. [CrossRef] [PubMed]
7. Gu, M.; Kong, H.-H. Improvement in Fine Manual Dexterity in Children with Spinal Muscular Atrophy Type 2 after Nusinersen Injection: A Case Series. *Children* **2021**, *8*, 1039. [CrossRef] [PubMed]
8. Weaver, M.S.; Yuroff, A.; Sund, S.; Hetzel, S.; Halanski, M.A. Quality of Life Outcomes According to Differential Nusinersen Exposure in Pediatric Spinal Muscular Atrophy. *Children* **2021**, *8*, 604. [CrossRef] [PubMed]
9. Halanski, M.A.; Hanna, R.; Bernatz, J.; Twedt, M.; Sund, S.; Patterson, K.; Noonan, K.J.; Schultz, M.; Schroth, M.K.; Sharafinski, M.; et al. Sagittal Plane Deformities in Children with SMA2 following Posterior Spinal Instrumentation. *Children* **2021**, *8*, 703. [CrossRef] [PubMed]
10. Huddar, A.; Polavarapu, K.; Preethish-Kumar, V.; Bardhan, M.; Unnikrishnan, G.; Nashi, S.; Vengalil, S.; Priyadarshini, P.; Kulanthaivelu, K.; Arunachal, G.; et al. Expanding the Phenotypic Spectrum of ECEL1-Associated Distal Arthrogryposis. *Children* **2021**, *8*, 909. [CrossRef] [PubMed]

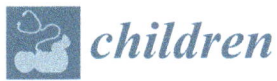

Review

Differential Diagnosis of Acquired and Hereditary Neuropathies in Children and Adolescents—Consensus-Based Practice Guidelines

Rudolf Korinthenberg [1,*], Regina Trollmann [2], Barbara Plecko [3], Georg M. Stettner [4], Markus Blankenburg [5], Joachim Weis [6], Benedikt Schoser [7], Wolfgang Müller-Felber [8], Nina Lochbuehler [9], Gabriele Hahn [10] and Sabine Rudnik-Schöneborn [11]

[1] Division of Neuropaediatrics and Muscular Disorders, Faculty of Medicine, University Medical Center (UMC), University of Freiburg, 79106 Freiburg, Germany
[2] Department of Pediatrics, Division of Neuropaediatrics, Friedrich-Alexander-Universität Erlangen-Nürnberg (FAU), 91054 Erlangen, Germany; regina.trollmann@uk-erlangen.de
[3] Department of Pediatrics and Adolescent Medicine, Medical University Graz, 8036 Graz, Austria; barbara.plecko@medunigraz.at
[4] Neuromuscular Center Zurich, Department of Pediatric Neurology, University Children's Hospital Zurich, University of Zurich, 8032 Zurich, Switzerland; georg.stettner@kispi.uzh.ch
[5] Department of Pediatric Neurology, Klinikum Stuttgart, Olgahospital, 70174 Stuttgart, Germany; m.blankenburg@klinikum-stuttgart.de
[6] Institute of Neuropathology, RWTH Aachen University Hospital, 52074 Aachen, Germany; jweis@ukaachen.de
[7] Friedrich-Baur-Institute, Department of Neurology, Ludwig-Maximilians-University of Munich, Ziemssenstr. 1a, 80336 Munich, Germany; benedikt.schoser@med.uni-muenchen.de
[8] Department of Neuropaediatrics, UMC, LMU Munich, 80337 Munich, Germany; wolfgang.mueller-felber@med.uni-muenchen.de
[9] Pediatric Radiology, Institute of Radiology, Olgahospital, Klinikum Stuttgart, 70174 Stuttgart, Germany; n.lochbuehler@klinikum-stuttgart.de
[10] Department of Radiological Diagnostics, UMC, University of Dresden, 01307 Dresden, Germany; gabrie-le.hahn@uniklinikum-dresden.de
[11] Division of Human Genetics, Medical University of Innsbruck, 6020 Innsbruck, Austria; sabine.rudnik@i-med.ac.at
* Correspondence: rudolf.korinthenberg@uniklinik-freiburg.de; Tel.: +49-761-46017

Abstract: Disorders of the peripheral nerves can be caused by a broad spectrum of acquired or hereditary aetiologies. The objective of these practice guidelines is to provide the reader with information about the differential diagnostic workup for a target-oriented diagnosis. Following an initiative of the German-speaking Society of Neuropaediatrics, delegates from 10 German societies dedicated to neuroscience worked in close co-operation to write this guideline. Applying the Delphi methodology, the authors carried out a formal consensus process to develop practice recommendations. These covered the important diagnostic steps both for acquired neuropathies (traumatic, infectious, inflammatory) and the spectrum of hereditary Charcot–Marie–Tooth (CMT) diseases. Some of our most important recommendations are that: (i) The indication for further diagnostics must be based on the patient's history and clinical findings; (ii) Potential toxic neuropathy also has to be considered; (iii) For focal and regional neuropathies of unknown aetiology, nerve sonography and MRI should be performed; and (iv) For demyelinated hereditary neuropathy, genetic diagnostics should first address PMP22 gene deletion: once that has been excluded, massive parallel sequencing including an analysis of relevant CMT-genes should be performed. This article contains a short version of the guidelines. The full-length text (in German) can be found at the Website of the "Arbeitsgemeinschaft der Wissenschftlichen Medizinischen Fachgesellschaften e.V. (AWMF), Germany.

Keywords: neuropathy; children; adolescents; Charcot–Marie–Tooth disease; traumatic neuropathy; inflammatory neuropathy; metabolic neuropathy

1. Introduction

Peripheral neuropathies are among the more frequent diseases confronting neurologists in their daily practice. The spectrum of aetiologies, clinical presentations, and disease courses is very broad, and differs considerably depending on the patient's age. Differential diagnostics for children and adolescents can be especially challenging because the more frequent neuropathies affecting adults (the diabetic, alcoholic, and vascular forms) very seldom (if at all) affect children, whereas rare hereditary and metabolic syndromes reveal a vast aetiological spectrum. This situation is made even more difficult because electrophysiological examination methods are often distressing for children, and only a few paediatricians are trained in electrophysiological methods.

These guidelines have been drafted for a wide variety of paediatricians and specialists (neuropaediatricians, neurologists and clinical neurophysiologists, genetic counsellors and consulting services, paediatric neuroradiologists, neuropathologists, and paediatric metabolic specialists) to provide orientation regarding diseases of the peripheral nerves affecting children and adolescents. The aim of these guidelines is to describe the state-of-the-art differential diagnoses and consensus-based target- and cost-oriented diagnostics.

2. Materials and Methods

The methods applied for these guidelines follow the regulations of the Arbeitsgemeinschaft der Wissenschaftlichen Medizinischen Fachgesellschaften (AWMF; Version 1.1, 27.02.2013) [1]. The basis for the present version of guidelines was a non-systematic review of the recent literature by the coordinating author and by the co-operating specialists for their respective fields of expertise. All these specialists also have vast practical experience in their fields, so their clinical perspectives in addition to economic aspects have enriched these guidelines. As the Delphi technique requires, the diagnostic recommendations were considered and consented to by the whole working group in a multi-step approach. In the first step, the coordinating author collated proposals from the group members, put them into written form, and returned them to the group. Each member could then agree to a recommendation or express another opinion to be discussed. Next, the coordinating author collected all the members' feedback and presented their discussion points in an anonymous form. Those were then sent back to the group members, who reconsidered each recommendation. This process was repeated until a solid consensus on each recommendation was achieved.

The power of a recommendation was classified in 3 levels, each with its own designation [1]:

- Strong recommendation: we recommend doing/recommend not doing
- Moderate recommendation: we suggest doing/suggest not doing
- Recommendation is open: may/can be done

The strength of consensus was classified as [1]:

- Strong consensus: >95% agreement of voters
- Consensus: >75–95% of voters
- Consent of majority: >50–75% of voters
- No consent of majority: <50% of voters

We achieved a "strong consensus" or "consensus" on all recommendations after the third round of consideration. Additionally, the text and comments of the guidelines were informally optimized by the guideline group through several voting sessions. Finally, the boards of all the participating scientific societies gave their final approval of the guidelines. The full-length text of the guidelines (in German) can be found at https://www.awmf.org/leitlinien/detail/ll/022-027.html (accessed on 6 August 2021).

3. Definition and Classification of Neuropathies in Children and Adolescents

Neuropathies are diseases of the peripheral and cranial nerves, whose anatomical and function-bearing structures consist of axons and myelin sheaths, endo-, peri-, and epineural connective tissue, and the vasa nervorum. Hereditary, traumatic, malignant, inflammatory, vascular, and metabolic disorders can cause damage to these structures. They can affect many nerves (polyneuropathy), or individual nerves (mononeuropathy, mononeuritis multiplex). Table 1 contains an overview.

Table 1. Survey of neuropathies in children and adolescents.

Hereditary Neuropathies	Acquired Neuropathies
1. **Hereditary Motor-Sensory Neuropathies (HMSN)/Charcot–Marie–Tooth (CMT) Neuropathies** CMT1 (demyelinating, AD) CMT2 (axonal, AD or AR) Intermediate CMT (AD or AR) CMT4 (demyelinating, AR) CMTX (demyelinating, axonal, XD, XR)	1. **Polyneuropathies** Inflammatory (infectious, postinfectious (GBS, CIDP), vasculitis) Toxic (drugs, heavy metals) Metabolic/malnutrition (uremia, diabetes, dysproteinemia, vitamin deficiency, hypervitaminoses) Paraneoplastic Critical-illness neuropathy Small-fibre neuropathy
2. **Hereditary Sensory-Autonomous Neuropathies (HSAN)** HSAN1 (AD) HSAN2-8 (AR)	2. **Mononeuritis multiplex** Inflammatory
3. **Hereditary Motor Neuropathies (HMN)** HMN (AD) DSMA (AR) DSMAX (XD)	3. **Mononeuropathies** Inflammatory Traumatic Nerve tumours Nerve compression syndromes
4. **Episodic Neuropathies** HNPP (AD) HNA (AD)	4. **Neuralgic shoulder amyotrophy, plexopathies** Traumatic Inflammatory
5. **Syndromic neuropathies** Neuropathies in the context of neurometabolic diseases Neuropathies in the context of neurodegenerative diseases	

DSMA: distal spinal muscular atrophy; HNPP: hereditary neuropathy with pressure palsies; HNA: hereditary neuralgic amyotrophy; AD: autosomal dominant; AR: autosomal recessive; XD: X-chromosomal-dominant; XR: X-chromosomal recessive. Comprehensive names for groups of diseases are printed in bold.

Nerve injuries occur due to sharp or dull mechanical effects or tearing. A functional conduction disorder without a transected axon is termed "neurapraxia", which heals relatively quickly. A transected axon (but with intact adjacent structures) is termed "axonotmesis". Here, recovery is usually achieved by sprouting from the proximal axon end. In cases of "neurotmesis", the entire nerve's continuity is broken, frequently resulting in a scar neuroma; here, a spontaneous re-innervation is unlikely to occur [2].

Acute para- and postinfectious neuropathies are most frequently observed in classic peripheral facial nerve paresis (idiopathic, or infectious through Borrelia burgdorferi and varicella-zoster virus), and in a generalized form as demyelinating or axonal Guillain–Barré syndrome (GBS). These are either caused by a direct invasion by the pathogen into nerves and the spinal ganglia accompanied by inflammatory infiltrates (i.e., herpes zoster, herpes simplex, lepromatous and tubercular lepra, various parasitic agents), vasculitis disorders (borreliosis, early symptomatic HIV infection), demyelination of Schwann cells (Guillain–Barré syndrome, diphtheria), or blocking of axonal transmission by antiganglioside antibodies (axonal forms of GBS: acute motor axonal neuropathy (AMAN), acute motor-sensory axonal neuropathy (AMSAN)).

Nongenetically caused metabolic polyneuropathies can affect children and adolescents, especially in conjunction with chronic kidney failure and diabetes mellitus [3,4]. Neuropathies caused by vitamin deficiencies occur through malnutrition, resorption disorders, and insufficient parenteral feeding via a shortage of vitamin B complex (B1, -2, -6, -12) and vitamin E [5]. The cause of critical illness-neuromyopathy occasionally diagnosed in ICU patients undergoing respirator treatment is unclear [6].

Toxic neuropathies can be caused by medical drugs, heavy metals, organic solvents, and organic phosphoric acid esters. Their pathophysiologies are generally associated with axonal damage affecting various cellular mechanisms [5,7].

Secondary neuropathies in association with collagenoses or vasculitis syndromes are extremely rare in children and adolescents. They usually occur as multiplex mononeuropathies and are pathologically characterised by segmental perivascular infiltrates and axonal lesions.

The non-syndromic hereditary neuropathies are clinically, genetically, pathologically, and electrophysiologically heterogeneous. The largest group among them, formerly called HMSN, is now classified according to the OMIM system and in reference to the neurologists who first described them as Charcot–Marie–Tooth (CMT) neuropathies, depending on their genetic causes. Neuropathologically speaking, they are differentiated according to what is primarily damaged—namely the axon, or myelin sheath [8]. The hereditary sensory-autonomic neuropathies (HSN) and hereditary motor neuropathies (HMN) could be regarded as CMT-related diseases with some similar features.

In addition to these isolated hereditary motor-sensory neuropathies, there is a broad range of disorders of the peripheral nerves in **complex neurometabolic and neurodegenerative diseases** revealing mainly CNS symptoms [9–11]. Here, usually the peripheral neuropathy manifests as a minor symptom, it is rarely the primary manifestation leading to diagnosis. Specific disease-related biochemical or histopathological findings are frequently associated with these diseases.

4. The Diagnostic Methods

4.1. History and Clinical Evaluation

Recommendation 1: Should a neuropathy be suspected, we recommend that a thorough patient history be taken, including the family's history. In addition to their known medical problems, information on previous infections and toxin exposures should be acquired.

Strength of consensus: strong (10/10)

Commentary: The patient history should incorporate the initial symptoms and the course, and exposure to potentially causative factors in the patient's past and family history. Early symptoms to ask for include neonatal and infantile muscular hypotonia and problems with sucking and swallowing, delayed motor development and walking, clumsiness and poor co-ordination compared to peers.

Recommendation 2: We recommend that a clinical examination include testing the patient's skin and muscle trophics, their strength or paresis grade, and their reflex and sensory status.

Strength of consensus: strong (10/10)

Commentary: Peripheral neuropathies usually manifest as muscle weakness, loss of deep tendon reflexes, and distal muscle atrophy. Foot deformities and other contractures result from muscular imbalance and frequently manifest as pes cavus and in severe cases as equinus or club foot. Typical neurological symptoms include an inability to walk on heels, steppage gait, and abnormal co-ordination in walking and manipulation (doing buttons, peg-in-hole tests). Sensory anomalies may also appear whereby the function of the large sensory fibres (touch, deep sensitivity) is usually more strongly affected than small-fibre function (pain and temperature sensations). Sensory ataxia with a positive Romberg sign may become apparent. Autonomous skin disorders (coldness, hypohidrosis, hyperhidrosis) as well as the regulation disorders caused by impaired autonomic nerve function (i.e., bladder emptying problems) can occur.

Recommendation 3: We recommend that the indication for more extensive diagnostics (electrophysiology, imaging, CSF diagnostics, lab work-up, toxicology, molecular genetics, biopsy) be determined depending strongly on the patient's medical history and clinical findings.

Strength of consensus: strong (10/10)

4.2. Electrophysiological Diagnostics

Clinical neurophysiology plays a key role in diagnosing neuropathies [12]. The most essential aspects to investigate when neuropathy is suspected are:

- Evidence or exclusion of peripheral nerve damage
- Identification of the affected structures (motor, sensory or sensorimotor neuropathy)
- Determination of the pathomechanism (axonal, demyelinating, or mixed damage)
- Any signs of florid denervation or re-innervation
- Signs of any additional involvement of CNS structures

It is essential that the diagnostic methods applied can be expected to yield information which extends beyond the patient's clinical findings. To spare children from unnecessary discomfort and worry, clinical and electrophysiological diagnostics must go hand in hand, and the physician needs to have the expertise and experience to ensure this [13,14]. Electrophysiological examinations, especially needle electromyography, are considered an invasive procedure. The examiner is assumed to possess not just knowledge of the age-specific normal values [15], but also a familiarity with the methods and psychological approaches young patients require. On suspicion of a dominantly inherited CMT it can make sense to investigate the parents instead of their young child.

Recommendation 4: We recommend that the electrophysiological diagnostics include motor and sensory neurographies. We suggest that the exam range be oriented along the concrete issues at hand and the patient's tolerance level.

Strength of consensus: strong (10/10)

Commentary: Motor and sensory neurographies help identify the neuropathies' fundamental pathomechanism, namely whether it is primarily demyelinating or axonal (Table 2). However, with some neuropathies, it is not possible to definitively differentiate between these (mixed types, intermediate types). If a compressed nerve or other circumscribed lesion is suspected, the clinician can attempt to localise the lesion by stimulating the nerves at different anatomical points along the nerve course (latency or amplitude jump, slowing in nerve conduction velocity (NCV) in the affected section, delayed distal motor latency). Most neuropathies in childhood also reveal obvious abnormalities in sensory neurography, for example, reduced amplitude in the sensory nerve action potentials (SNAP) and possibly a slower NCV. A normal sensory neurography in a patient with purely motor symptoms should make the physician consider dHMN or DSMA.

Table 2. Electrophysiological criteria for demyelinating or axonal damage to peripheral nerves.

	Motor Neurography	EMG
Demyelination	Slowing of NCV, prolongation of distal-motor latency, prolongated or deficient F-waves (in proximal demyelination), abnormal dispersion of CMAP and partial conduction block (acquired multifocal demyelination, for example CIDP)	Normal findings when axonal anomalies are absent
Axonal damage	Lowered CMAP amplitude (can also be due to muscular atrophy/myopathy)	Florid denervation: fibrillation potentials, positive sharp waves, reduced interference pattern Chronic denervation with re-innervation: abnormal high-amplitude and polyphasic potentials, reduced interference pattern

NCV: nerve conduction velocity; CMAP: compound muscle action potential.

Recommendation 5: We suggest that the patient undergo electromyography when seeking signs of denervation as evidence for an acute or chronic axonal neuropathy, or when there is a suspicion of an accompanying or alternative myopathy.

Strength of consensus: strong (10/10)

Commentary: An EMG is advisable when clarifying a neuropathy diagnosis to detect axonal lesions, i.e., for a case of acute axonal GBS, a CMT with a normal NCV, and to differentially distinguish a neuropathy from distal spinal muscle atrophy or myopathy (Table 2). This enables an assessment of pathologic spontaneous activity (positive sharp waves, fibrillations), the discharge and recruiting pattern of motor units, and the configuration of motor unit potentials (MUP). There is also an indication when seeking for signs of re-innervation, especially following traumatic neuropathy [2]. In addition, myotonic and neuromyotonic discharges can be useful in detecting diseases with muscular or nerve hyperexcitability.

Recommendation 6: We suggest that visual and/or acoustically evoked potentials be examined in case of a systemic disease involving the peripheral and central nervous system.
Strength of consensus: strong (10/10)
Commentary: The examination of visual and auditory evoked potentials enables us to assess the functionality of these specific peripheral and central sensory pathways. However, the investigation of somatosensory-evoked potentials (SEP) often fails or is inconclusive because of peripheral nerve damage. Nonetheless, with a high number of stimulations, a central summation effect can sometimes result in a recordable SEP.

4.3. Sensory and Vegetative Functional Diagnostics

Recommendation 7: Should isolated small-fibre neuropathy be suspected, quantitative sensory testing can be performed.
Strength of consensus: consensus (8/10)
Commentary: Neuropathies affecting the thin or non-myelinated (Aδ- and C-) fibres necessary for pain and temperature sensation (small-fibre neuropathy) also occur in childhood and adolescence. However, they are often detected at a late stage or not at all because of their vague or uncharacteristic clinical symptoms such as pain, fatigue, and nausea. Auto-immune disorders, adolescent-onset Morbus Fabry and familial amyloid polyneuropathy (FAP), or other hereditary sensory neuropathies are known causes [16,17]. While routine electroneurography does not usually help diagnostically, the functional disturbance can be detected via quantitative sensory testing (QST). QST has been validated for children aged 6 years and beyond, but it is currently available mainly in pain clinics [3]. However, to objectively diagnose a small-fibre neuropathy or FAP, a skin biopsy and genetic testing is ultimately required [16,17] (see also neuropathology).

Recommendation 8: In case of suspected autonomic neuropathy, examinations to detect an autonomic function disorder can be performed (i.e., heart rate variability, sympathetic skin reactions, and the tilt-table test).
Strength of consensus: strong (10/10)
Commentary: The autonomic nervous system should be examined, for example in case of severe GBS and hereditary autonomous neuropathies to estimate the risk of heart arrhythmias and/or cardiac arrest. This examination is available in paediatric and adult cardiology departments [18].

4.4. Imaging Diagnostics

Recommendation 9: We recommend imaging procedures (ultrasound and MRI) for cases of local or regional neuropathies without a definitive aetiological explanation; imaging methods could reveal possible therapy-relevant lesions (nerve tumour, nerve entrapment syndrome, focal inflammation).
Strength of consensus: strong (10/10)
Commentary: Clinical neurological examinations are now enhanced by imaging technologies. The discovery of a causative tumour or compression enables surgery to de-compress the nerve.

Recommendation 10: In cases of polyneuropathies and diffuse neuropathies with doubtful clinical-electrophysiological findings and an indication to rule out an intraspinal or radicular tumour or prolapsed disc, we recommend MRI imaging or ultrasound.

Strength of consensus: strong (10/10)

Recommendation 11: Imaging via spinal MRI or ultrasound of the proximal nerves may also be performed to detect anomalies typical of inflammatory diseases (GBS, CIDP) in case the patient's findings so far have been inconclusive.

Strength of consensus: strong (10/10)

Commentary: In patients with Guillain–Barré syndrome, CIDP, and other inflammatory radiculopathies, the spinal MRI often reveals thickening and contrast-medium enhancement in the spinal and cranial nerve roots [19–21]. Examinations of circumscribed and diffuse lesions and diseases of the nerve plexus and peripheral nerves via high-resolution nerve MRI or sonography are highly interesting [22–24]. However, as with electrophysiology, sonographic examinations of the peripheral, proximal, and cerebral nerves require a great deal of expertise and experience and are only available in few paediatric neurology and/or neuromuscular expert centres, making a general recommendation in these guidelines premature at this time.

4.5. Laboratory and Other Paraclinical Diagnostics

Laboratory parameters (Table 3) enable us to clarify secondary neuropathies induced by primary internal diseases (liver or kidney diseases, diabetes, collagenoses). If there are hints of a disease caused by a vitamin deficiency, the corresponding analyses should be undertaken, as in case a neurometabolic disorder in suspected [11].

Table 3. Laboratory tests for clinically and electrophysiologically suspicious cases.

Disorder	Lab Diagnostics
Infectious neuropathy	Serology and possible swabs, *Borrelia burgdorferi*, VZV, etc.
Inflammatory systemic diseases	ESR, CRP, ANA, double-stranded DNS-ab, C3 complement, ACE, lysozymes, immunoelectrophoretis, cryoglobulin
GBS, CIDP	CSF protein, CSF cell count, pathogen serology (CMV, *Mycopl. pneumoniae*, *Campylobacter jejuni*), anti-gangliosid antibodies (seldom positive), antibodies against paranodal proteins (neurofascin, etc.)
M. Refsum and other peroxisomopathies	Phytanic acid, VLCFA in serum
Bassen–Kornzweig syndrome (a-betalipoproteinemia)	Electrophoresis, lipid electrophoresis, vitamin E
Primary vitamin E resorption disorder	Vitamin E
Secondary vitamin resorption disorders	Vitamin D (Ca, P, AP, parathormone), vitamin E, vitamin K (INR, quick value), folic acid, vitamin B12 (with holotranscobalamin and methylmalonic acid), thiamin, riboflavin. Vitamin B6 (overdose?)
CDG syndromes	Isoelectric transferrin focussing
Metachromatic leukodystrophy and M. Krabbe	CSF protein, lysosomal enzymes
Mitochondriopathies	Lactate in plasma and CSF, possible muscle biopsy for biochemical analyses

4.6. Neuropathological Diagnostics

Recommendation 12: We recommend performing a nerve biopsy in case the diagnosis of a severe or progressing polyneuropathy is not otherwise possible, that is, via less invasive methods, and provided a firm diagnosis and therapy can be the consequence. This applies mainly to patients suspected of having vasculitis.

Strength of consensus: strong (10/10)

Commentary: Determining the indication for a nerve biopsy cannot be taken lightly; it requires great caution and differentiation. It is particularly significant for differential diagnostic workup when neuropathies are being considered that are not hereditary and can be effectively treated. In these categories belong infections such as vasculitis and perineuritis, as well as atypically presenting inflammatory neuropathies (chronic inflammatory demyelinating or axonal neuropathy), nerves compromised by a lymphoma, and amyloid neuropathy [25,26]. Histological tests are generally done in the sensory sural nerve and require a compression-free section of the nerve. A part thereof is fixed in formalin for paraffin histology including Congo red or thioflavin-staining and immunohistochemistry; the other is fixed in glutaraldehyde (embedding in synthetic resin for semi-thin section/toluidine blue-staining and possible electron microscopy) [27]. Nerve biopsies should only be carried out and analysed in highly specialised centres; collecting adequate tissue from infants is extremely difficult and requires a very experienced surgeon [28].

Suspected inherited sensory neuropathy or small-fibre neuropathy (SFN) calls for a **skin punch biopsy** including immunohistochemistry of epidermal and dermal nerve fibres with staining for Protein Gene Product 9.5 (PGP9.5); it also allows the study of dermal myelinated fibres, autonomic innervation (sweat glands, arrector pili muscle, arterio-venous anastomosis), and mechanoreceptors. It is a less invasive procedure used to obtain diagnosis, but it also requires expertise and the knowledge of norm values appropriate to the given age group [17,29]. Adolescent-onset FAP can be suspected by the presentation of amyloid deposits but needs genetic testing of the TTR gene for confirmation [16].

4.7. Genetic Diagnostics

Recommendation 13: In the case of suspected hereditary neuropathy we recommend molecular genetic diagnostics which include different methods depending on the patient's clinical findings and family's medical history.

Strength of consensus: strong (10/10)

Comment: Over 100 genes have been reported as being responsible for causing CMT neuropathies. The diagnostic algorithm depends on multiple factors of the presenting patient. If the family is known to carry a specific mutation, that can be verified in the patient via MLPA or Sanger sequencing. If CMT neuropathy is suspected without a known mutation, the first diagnostic step should be to identify the PMP22 gene's copy number (usually via MLPA), especially in the case of demyelinating polyneuropathy. If that result is inconspicuous, massive parallel sequencing (next-generation sequencing (NGS)) is currently usually carried out, as it enables the most rapid and cost-effective analysis of many genes [8].

The **Gene Diagnostics Law** (GenDG) has been in effect in Germany since 2010. It mandates that special measures be taken to ensure that patients are well-informed before consenting to such tests. While any physician can schedule and carry out diagnostic examinations in patients with symptoms, the use of predictive genetic tests in healthy persons who carry a risk or in individuals with a possible genetic predisposition must be preceded by genetic counselling, which must only be conducted by certified physicians qualified to engage in genetic counselling and consultation. The genetic counselling must also include the information that molecular analysis may bring to light additional findings from genome diagnostics raising entirely different issues such as a hereditary cancer risk or risk for other neurological diseases.

5. Differential Diagnosis of Acquired and Hereditary Neuropathies in Children and Adolescents

5.1. Nerve Injuries

Recommendation 14: If peripheral nerve injury is suspected, we recommend a clinical examination to locate the affected nerve and lesion site, and to supplement this if needed by a neurophysiological investigation.

Strength of consensus: strong (10/10)

Commentary: Some injured or malfunctioning nerves are clinically practically impossible to identify; they can only be objectively assessed electrophysiologically (i.e., weakness in the palmar hand muscles with a failing pre-load in radial paresis) [2].

Recommendation 15: We recommend a liberal indication to perform imaging (especially ultrasound) diagnostics in patients with a nerve lesion, particularly when operative treatment is likely necessary (i.e., neuronotmesis, nerve compression in a fracture gap, compression by a haematoma or tumour).

Strength of consensus: strong (10/10)

Commentary: Lesions affecting individual nerves or nerve plexus are often caused by typical accidents or traumas. Their clinical symptoms depend on the function of the affected nerve (motor-sensory mixed) and on the lesion's location. An entirely transected nerve leads to paralysis of the innervated musculature, loss of sensation, and when the N. medianus and tibialis are transected, to the loss of sweat secretion in that region. Should the patient reveal some remaining function, the likelihood of continuity and spontaneous recuperation rises. Table 4 illustrates the main postnatal lesions and their motor and sensory symptoms as well as their most frequent causes.

Table 4. Clinical appearance and aetiology of peripheral nerve lesions.

Site of Lesion	Motor Defect	Sensory Defect	Aetiologies
Upper brachial plexus	Shoulder abduction and external rotation, elbow flexion, supination	Lateral/radial arm from shoulder to metacarpo-phalangeal joint of thumb	Strain/tearing of the shoulder, perinatal trauma, neuralgic amyotrophy, serogenetic neuritis, tumour infiltration
Lower brachial plexus	Finger and wrist flexion, finger ab- and -adduction, possibly Horner syndrome	Axillary and ulnar side of the arm from elbow to hand and finger IV and V	Trauma as above, abnormal cervical rib, scalenus syndrome, tumour infiltration
Long thoracic nerve	Elevation and rotation of scapula, winged scapula on shoulder flexion	-	»back packer palsy«, neuralgic amyotrophy
Radial nerve	Extension of wrist and metacarpo-phalangeal joints, abduction of thumb, extension of thumb and finger II (»flaccid drop of the hand«)	Back of the hand overlying metacarpals I and II	Humerus shaft fracture, pressure palsy
Median nerve	Flexion of wrist, flexion of finger I–III (»Schwurhand«)	Volar side of the hand and fingers I to the radial side of IV, dorsal side of same fingers	Supracondylar fracture of humerus, pressure palsy, carpal tunnel syndrome
Ulnar nerve	Flexion of wrist and metacarpo-phalangeal joint IV–V, ab-/adduction III–V, thumb adduction (»Krallenhand«)	Volar and dorsal side of hand and fingers IV and V (not radial side finger IV)	Supracondylar fracture of humerus, elbow fracture, pressure palsy
Ischiadic nerve	Combination of tibial- and peroneal lesion	Combination of tibial- and peroneal lesion	Ischiadic lesion at misplaced injection, pelvic fractures
Tibial nerve	Foot- and toe flexors, loss of Achilles tendon reflex	Plantar side of the foot, lateral side of the foot	Fractures, injury to the hollow of the knee
Peroneal nerve	Foot extension (»Steppage gait«)	Lateral lower leg, back of the foot	Fibular fracture, pressure palsy

Recommendation 16: Electrophysiological tests can be done repeatedly to follow up patients and keep track of denervation and re-innervation processes, thus enabling a more accurate prognosis after a nerve lesion.

Strength of consensus: strong (10/10)

Commentary: A nerve's continuity can be confirmed via electrophysiological tests in patients suffering from total clinical paralysis following a nerve lesion. For patients who fail to fully recover after a nerve trauma, we suggest electrophysiological controls at 3-month intervals to evaluate the extent and direction of re-innervation, as they yield such information earlier than clinical examinations can [2].

5.2. Mononeuritis, Mononeuritis Multiplex

Recommendation 17: We recommend brain MR imaging in case of a suspected non-idiopathic facial nerve palsy; this is especially recommended in case of multiple cranial nerve lesions.

Strength of consensus: strong (10/10)

Recommendation 18: We recommend that infectiological blood tests be run for clinically suspected cases of borreliosis to confirm the aetiology; we suggest a lumbar puncture and cell count as well as serological tests in CSF be carried out to diagnose CNS involvement.

Strength of consensus: consensus (9/10)

Commentary: A peripheral or nuclear lesion of the facial nerve leads to paralysis in the mimic muscles innervated by all three of its branches. In contrast, a lesion in the corticobulbar tract leaves the function of the frontal branch intact thanks to bilateral cortical representation. Depending on where it is located, a nerve lesion along the facial canal in the base of the skull can cause lacrimal secretion to fail, as well as a loss the stapedius-reflex with hyperakusis and a loss of taste sensation on the affected side. Isolated facial paresis in childhood is usually idiopathic and inflammatory (Bell's palsy). However, during the summer and autumn, cases of facial paresis are frequently caused by neuroborreliosis. It is often accompanied by minor symptoms of meningeal irritation; mononuclear CSF pleocytosis is detected in over 90% of such cases. The presence of pleocytosis and elevated Borrelia antibody titers in the CSF are required as evidence of neurological involvement [30]. Other causes of facial nerve palsy are zoster oticus, otitis media, petrosal bone fractures, and tumours in the brain stem and cerebello-pontine angle [31].

Further infectious forms of neuritis are manifested in the context of specific infections (borreliosis, zoster, diphtheria, leprosy). These can strongly determine each disease's presentation, or go largely undetected as secondary phenomena. Their clinical symptoms are focal or multifocal, and cranial nerves are often affected. Cases of symmetric polyneuritis are seldom: in that case, it can be difficult to differentiate these from a post-infectious Guillain–Barré syndrome.

Recommendation 19: In cases of suspected vasculitis neuropathy, we recommend a biopsy if a firm diagnosis has proven impossible with other less invasive methods (for example, to detect typical antibodies).

Strength of consensus: strong (10/10)

Commentary: Cranial or spinal neuropathies or mononeuritis multiplex can appear in conjunction with different inflammatory systemic diseases. They can occur in lupus erythematodes, polyarteriitis nodosa, granulomatosis associated with polyangiitis Wegener, eosinophilic granulomatosis associated with polyangiitis Churg–Strauss, Boeck' disease, Schönlein–Henoch syndrome, inflammatory intestinal disorders, and other autoimmune diseases [32,33]. Guillain–Barré syndrome may also be present in conjunction with these illnesses, an important factor to consider in terms of the different therapeutic consequences.

5.3. Guillain–Barré Syndrome (GBS) and Chronic Inflammatory Demyelinating Polyneuropathy (CIDP)

We recommend consulting the corresponding S3 guidelines for the diagnosis and treatment of acute **GBS**, whose progressive phase is limited to 4 weeks [34]. CIDP has to be assumed if a patient exhibits a longer protracted, progressing, or fluctuating disease course.

Recommendation 20: In the case of prolonged demyelinating polyneuropathy revealing an obviously fluctuating or progressing course we recommend diagnostics for a suspected CIDP (including a CSF protein and cell count, possibly also a spinal MRI); we also recommend therapy attempts involving intravenous immunoglobulin (IvIG), plasmapheresis, or corticosteroids for inconclusive cases.

Strength of consensus: strong (10/10)

Commentary: CIDP can affect all age groups. Unlike acute GBS, CIDP exhibits a chronic, continuous or stepwise progressing or relapsing–remitting course. Paediatric diagnostic criteria for CIDP mandate a progressing period lasting at least 4 weeks. However, up to 20% begin as acute GBS (aCIDP) and move from there to a chronic or relapsing course [35,36]. The clinical symptoms consist of motor and sensory impairments, where the impairment of just one function is more seldom. The neuropathy is usually symmetrically distributed, primarily in the distal legs. However, the symptoms can first appear in the arms and involve the neck muscles. The cranial nerves are often affected; however, respiratory insufficiency is less frequent than in patients with GBS. Additional diagnostic criteria comprise increased CSF protein in conjunction with a normal cell count, as well as an electrophysiological proof of multiple segmentally demyelinated nerves. Infectious, toxic, or metabolic neuropathies and a CNS process entailing a distinct sensory level and a paralysed sphincter must be ruled out. A high percentage of these patients lose the ability to walk unaided. The disease can last for months or many years [35–37]. Potentially effective therapies for CIDP are IvIG, plasmapheresis, or prednisolone of adequate duration (i.e., at least 3 months).

Recommendation 21: For patients with CIDP who are resistant to treatment with IvIG, plasmapheresis, and steroids, we recommend considering and testing for potential antibodies to paranodal proteins. We also recommend the patient to be re-examined for a potential hereditary aetiology (CMT). From adolescence onwards, familial amyloid polyneuropathy has to be considered, as it is frequently misrecognized as CIDP in the beginning [16].

Strength of consensus: strong (10/10)

Commentary: For children presenting a therapy-resistant and protracted course of a demyelinating polyneuropathy, we propose considering the possibility of a causation through antibodies to paranodal proteins like neurofascin-155; these "paranodopathies" may respond to rituximab even when the patient is IvIG-resistant [38–40]. Very slowly progressing CIDP is easily mistaken for a subacute course of **hypo- or demyelinating CMT**, and vice versa [41]. Increased CSF protein and excessive contrast medium absorption in the nerve roots on a spinal MRI are typical of CIDP, but neither is specific, and both can also accompany hereditary CMT neuropathies.

5.4. Toxic Neuropathies

Recommendation 22: We recommend that, in children also, the possibility of a toxic neuropathy always be considered. This can usually be ruled out by taking a careful patient history and ensuring the child undergoes a thorough clinical-electrophysiological examination. Specific laboratory investigations are rarely needed.

Strength of consensus: strong (10/10)

Commentary: A partial list of potential neurotoxic substances is found in Table 5.

Table 5. Toxic agents associated with polyneuropathy (selection).

Drugs	Heavy Metals and Solvents
Vincristin, cis-platinum	Lead
Taxane, epothilone	Gold
Bortezomib	Thallium
Thalidomide	Arsenic
Nitrofurantoin, isoniazid (INH)	Mercury
Hydantoine	n-Hexane
Chloramphenicol, metronidazol	Methyl-n-butylketone
Amphotericin	Triorthocresylphosphate

5.5. Hereditary Non-Syndromic Neuropathies in Children and Adolescents

5.5.1. Hereditary Motor-Sensory Neuropathies (HMSN), Charcot–Marie–Tooth (CMT)-Neuropathy

Clinical Presentations of CMT Neuropathies

The clinical evidence of **classic CMT neuropathy** consists of symmetric weakness and atrophy in the distal leg muscles, weak deep tendon reflexes, and a neurogenic talipes cavus. The disease's range of expression is extremely wide. These neuropathies usually become apparent in the **first** two decades of life. Most of their subtypes progress only slightly. Symptoms can spread to the thigh and hand musculature years later. Many of those affected exhibit few symptoms even in old age and are not detected until the family is screened. Yet, other individuals in the same family can present with early generalised weakness and suffer a very severe course.

The most frequent type of CMT is **CMT1**, the **demyelinating type.** It can be detected electrophysiologically, showing a homogeneously slowed motor nerve conduction velocity (NCV) of <38 m/s in the arm nerves (with the median nerve as reference nerve). The **axonal variant** of CMT neuropathy (**CMT2**) cannot be differentiated clinically from the demyelinating type; however, overlapping and mixed forms often make confirming a specific diagnosis very difficult. The situation is similar with **CMTX, the X-chromosomal dominant variant**, which is clinically usually apparent in males as CMT1, and in females often as axonal or mixed demyelinating-axonal neuropathy. **Additional symptoms** like hearing loss, optic atrophy, vocal cord paralysis, conspicuously rapid progression, atypical patterns in how the pareses are distributed, scoliosis, or renal insufficiency are potential signs of certain gene mutations [42,43].

Congenital HMSN/CMT neuropathies first becoming obvious in infancy are very rare, but nevertheless relevant for the paediatric neurologist. Because of their typical findings, these diseases used to be categorised as congenital hypomyelinating polyneuropathy and Déjerine–Sottas syndrome (previously CMT3) with demyelinating and hypertrophic neuropathy, pronounced sensory impairments, increased CSF protein, and a severe course. Molecular genetic evidence has shown that these are not independent genetic entities, but rather the clinically most severe manifestations of known phenotypically highly variable CMT mutations [44].

Episodic neuropathies are difficult to diagnose accurately because of their on–off phases. The most important form is autosomal-dominant **hereditary neuropathy with pressure palsies** (HNPP), with a prevalence of 7–16 individuals out of 100,000. This is characterised by recurring functional focal deficits in the peripheral nerves, especially at certain anatomically critical pressure points. It can develop over time into a chronic CMT1 or CMT2. Autosomal dominantly inherited **hereditary neuralgic amyotrophy** (HNA) is a further disease, which is characterised by burning shoulder pain and later, muscle atrophy.

Genetic Diagnostics for CMT Neuropathies

It is much more successful to confirm a genetic diagnosis of CMT1 (50–80% of all CMT patients) than of CMT2 (10–30% of patients). According to larger studies following comparable protocols, we can genetically identify the four most frequent genes (PMP22, GJB1/Cx32, MPZ/P0, MFN2) in 40–60% of patients in whom an inherited neuropathy is suspected [8]. In patients with CMT1A, PMP22 duplication is detected in 50–70% of cases, GJB1/Cx32 mutations in 9–18%, and MPZ/P0 mutations in 3–10%. The study results are more variable in patients with CMT2: GJB1/Cx32 in 7–19%, MFN2 in 2–20%, and MPZ/P0 in 1–6% of cases. The most frequent genes associated with autosomal-recessive CMT types are GDAP1 and SH3TC2. Mutations in GDAP1 are the most prevalent finding in autosomal dominant and recessive CMT2 cases in Spain and South Italy [45,46]. The HINT1 gene is especially prevalent in eastern Europe (Czech Republic); its clinical presentation is that of an axonal neuropathy accompanied by neuromyotony [8].

Recommendation 23: We recommend molecular-genetic diagnostics in case of a suspected demyelinating CMT neuropathy, starting by determining the number of PMP22 copies. This can also be done as the initial diagnostic step in case of an axonal CMT neuropathy.

Strength of consensus: consensus (9/10)

Commentary: Quantitative analysis of the PMP22 gene via MLPA to detect deletions and duplications is a rapid, reliable test method, while these larger duplications and deletions are not detected via NGS and Sanger sequencing. PMP22 duplications are identified in 50–70% of CMT1 patients. PMP22 deletions seldom also manifest as axonal CMT: CMT2 was clinically diagnosed in 1% of a series of 334 patients with PMP22 deletions.

This PMP22 deletion, however, amounted to 5.3% of the group with genetically proven CMT2 (n = 57), making it the fourth most frequent CMT2 aetiology [47].

Recommendation 24: Should an HNPP be suspected, we recommend (once a PMP22 deletion has been ruled out) analyses seeking intragenic PMP22 mutations.

Strength of consensus: strong (10/10)

Commentary: HNPP is characterised by mainly heterozygotic deletions of the PMP22 gene; loss-of-function point mutations in the PMP22 gene are found more seldom.

Recommendation 25: After ruling out PMP22 duplication or deletion, we recommend performing massive parallel sequencing of gene candidates when CMT neuropathy is suspected.

Strength of consensus: strong (10/10)

Commentary: It is expected that advances in genetic testing will identify more and more genes in which mutations lead to ultra-rare hereditary conditions including neuropathies, and that the frequency of causative mutations will be better defined via high-throughput technologies which enable numerous genes to be examined simultaneously. The most up-to-date information on the genes associated with neuropathies is found in the Online Mendelian Inheritance in Man data base (OMIM, www.ncbi.nlm.nih.gov/omim (accessed on 6 August 2021)). The US National Institutes of Health/NIH also provide an overview of genetic diagnostics for HMSN/CMT in their gene reviews (http://www.ncbi.nlm.nih.gov/books/NBK1358/ (accessed on 6 August 2021)).

5.5.2. Distal Hereditary Motor Neuropathies (dHMN)

This is a rare and genetically heterogeneous group of diseases characterised by exclusively motor symptoms affecting the distal muscle groups. Muscle atrophies and pareses primarily affect the lower extremities, but there are also forms more likely to affect the arm and hand muscles. There is some clinical and genetic overlap with distal spinal muscle atrophies that by electrophysiological and histological definition reveal no pathology in the peripheral nerves and exhibit neurogenic re-organisation in the affected musculature. dHMN can also overlap with spastic paraplegia (e.g., BSCL2). Thus, clinicians should pay attention to pyramidal signs and eventually perform motor evoked potentials.

Recommendation 26: We recommend performing massive parallel sequencing of gene candidates if a dHMN is suspected. PMP22 copies can be quantified beforehand.

Strength of consensus: consensus (9/10)

Commentary: The genetic clarification of dHMN/DSMA has improved greatly through high-throughput technologies in the last few years, and now lies in the range of 30–40% [48]. Because of dHMN's clinical and genetic overlapping with axonal CMT neuropathy, the genetic diagnostics are usually done simultaneously (Figures 1 and 2).

5.5.3. Hereditary Sensory and Autonomous Neuropathies (HSAN, HSN)

This group of extremely rare hereditary polyneuropathies is referred to as HSAN or HSN. It is primarily characterised by distally pronounced sensory-functional impairments and autonomic symptoms, and much less by minor motor impairments. Its classification in five different types becomes that much harder to follow the faster and more specifically new genes are being identified [49,50].

The autosomal-dominantly inherited **HSAN I types** usually become apparent in the second decade of life and begin with pain and impaired temperature sensation. Patients later suffer from the loss of other sensory capacities and spontaneous pain. The loss of sensory innervation triggers trophic anomalies and ulcers on the hands and feet, and not seldom gives rise to osteomyelitis and osteolysis. Less important are autonomic functional disorders (like excessive perspiration). **HSAN II–V** is inherited autosomal-recessively and usually first manifests in infancy or childhood; **HSAN II** is characterised by painless injuries (through the loss of sensation) and acrodystrophy and joint degeneration. **HSAN III** is also known as Riley–Day syndrome or familial dysautonomia; it causes autonomic-regulation impairments, vomiting, and primarily psychomotor retardation. **HSAN IV**'s dominant features are generalised anhidrosis accompanied by episodic bouts of fever already during infancy (CIPA) together with the loss of pain sensations and cognitive deficits. Children with **HSAN V** reveal no cognitive deficits, but otherwise a clinical presentation resembling that of HSAN IV [49].

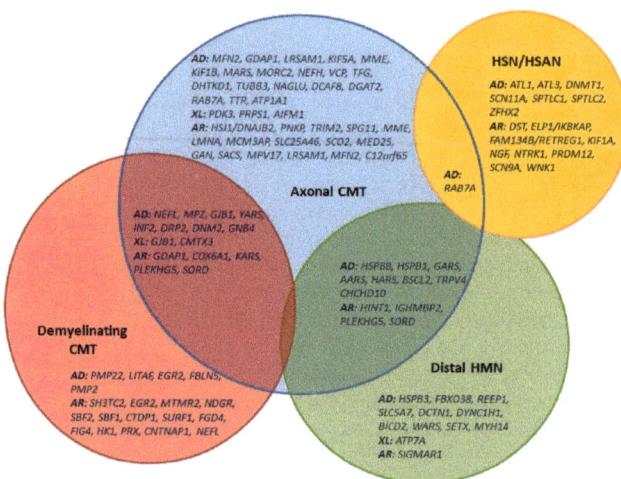

Figure 1. VENN diagram showing the distribution of mutations among clinical and electrophysiological groups of hereditary neuropathies (CMT/HSAN/dHMN) [8].

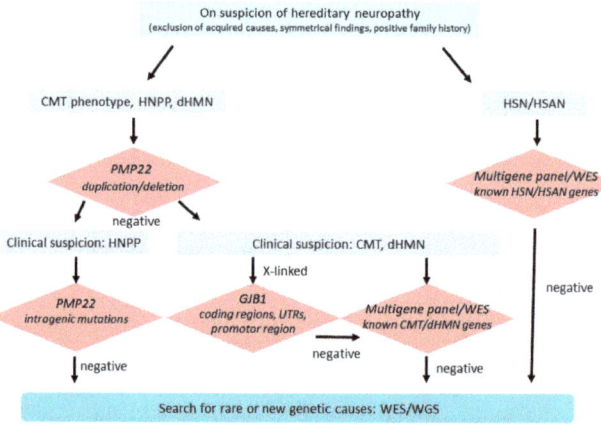

Figure 2. Algorithm to perform a genetic diagnosis of hereditary neuropathies [8].

Recommendation 27: Molecular genetic diagnostics via massive parallel sequencing of gene candidates is recommended to clarify cases of a suspected HSN/HSAN (see Figure 1).

Strength of consensus: strong (10/10)

Commentary: According to the very latest evidence, the responsible gene defects are only detected in 10–20% of families affected by HSAN/HSN [49,50]. As of the time these guidelines were compiled, no large investigations had been conducted targeting multi-gene panels or examination sequencing in association with this very rare group of diseases.

5.5.4. Genetic Diagnostic Algorithms

To decide which genes should be analysed to clarify the aetiology of a suspected hereditary neuropathy, it is first important to clinically specify the disease as CMT neuropathy, episodic neuropathy, purely motor dHMN, purely sensory HSN/HSAN, or neuropathy in the context of a multi-system disease (Figure 2).

A quantitative procedure (MLPA) is initially recommended in the case of suspected demyelinating CMT neuropathy or HNPP to identify the frequent PMP22 duplication or deletions (Figure 2). While this diagnostic approach will fail in case of HSAN, for axonal CMT or dHMN it can be performed, although with less expectation of a positive result than in CMT1/HNPP. If the MLPA finding is negative, massive parallel sequencing of gene candidates is nowadays standard for nearly all hereditary neuropathies.

As the four most frequent genes (PMP22, GJB1/Cx32, MPZ/P0, MFN2) are detected in 90–95% of positively genetically screened patients belonging to cohorts of mainly middle-European heritage [8], clinicians are justified to first have these genes assessed after clinical and thorough formal genetic differentiation before expanding their genetic investigation to detect rare genes.

Recommendation 28: If an X-chromosomal CMT neuropathy is suspected, we recommend analysis of the GJB1 gene including coding regions, untranslated regions (UTRs), and promoter regions.

Strength of consensus: strong (10/10)

Commentary: 10–15% of patients with an X-chromosomal CMT reveal GJB1 mutations in non-coding regions that cannot be detected via high-throughput sequencing (Figure 2).

As soon as a genetic diagnosis has been made, the affected family should be offered genetic counselling.

5.6. Peripheral Neuropathies Associated with Complex Genetic Diseases

Recommendation 29: Should a systemic neurodegenerative or metabolic disorder be suspected in a patient with polyneuropathy, we recommend that primarily those diseases for which there are effective therapies be ruled out.

Strength of consensus: strong (10/10)

Commentary: Peripheral neuropathies can also occur in a complex array of symptoms caused by a large number of different neurometabolic and neurodegenerative syndromes. Thanks to the progress made recently in genetic diagnostics, their numbers have risen dramatically. In their systematic review, Rossor et al. [11] describe over 150 genetically defined diseases. Only a small proportion of these are manifested in childhood, and many have only been described in one or a handful of families. The neuropathy is often just one aspect of a given disease, although it can cause the main symptoms for some time during the disease's initial stage. For a given genetic disease, the neuropathy may present as an isolated symptom in adulthood if the mutation's effect is weak; but children whose gene is largely dysfunctional usually suffer from progressive CNS deterioration and early death. It is significant to note that effective therapies are available for some of these diseases provided they are diagnosed early enough, which is why they must not be diagnostically overlooked (Table 6).

Table 6. Neuropathies in the context of complex hereditary diseases amenable to treatment [11].

Disease	Diagnostics	Treatment
Refsum syndrome	Axonal or demyelinated NP, phytanic acid, pristanic acid	Phytanic acid-restricted diet, plasmapheresis
Adrenoleukodystrophy	VLCFA	Presymptomatic BMT
Metachromatic leukodystrophy	Demyelinated NP, lysosomal enzymes	Presymptomatic BMT
Vitamin E malabsorption	Vitamin E in serum	Vitamin E
Bassen–Kornzweig syndrome	Abetalipoproteinemia	Vitamin E

Table 6. Cont.

Disease	Diagnostics	Treatment
B12 deficiencies in resorption and utilisation	Vit B12 in serum, methylmalonic acis, homocystein in serum	Vitamin B12
Folate deficiencies in resorption and utilisation	Folate, 5-Methyltetrahydrofolate	Folate, folinic acid
Cerebrotendinous xanthomatosis	Plasma cholestanol	Diet, chenodesoxycholic acid
Brown–Vialetto-van Laere syndrome	Bulbar paralysis, deafness, riboflavin in serum	Riboflavin
CD59 mutation	Anemia, paroxysmal nocturnal hematuria, relapsing NP	Eculizumab
Acute intermittent porphyria	Porphobilinogen	Glucose, haematin
Pyruvate dehydrogenase deficiency	Lactate, enzyme diagnostics, genetics	Ketogenic diet
Morbus Fabry (alpha-galactosidase A deficiency)	Severe acroparesthesias, autonomous neuropathy, angiokeratoma, corneal dystrophy, cardiovascular disease, stroke, renal impairment	Enzyme replacement therapy with agalsidase alfa or agalsidase beta
Familial amyloid polyneuropathy (onset from adolescence)	Symmetric sensory-motor and autonomic neuropathy, family history of neuropathy and/or cardiomyopathy, gi involvement, weight loss, carpal tunnel syndrome, TTR genetics	Liver transplantation, TTR stabilizers and gene modifying approaches in preparation [16]

BMT: bone marrow transplantation; VLCFA: very long-chain fatty acids; gi: gastrointestinal.

A list of relevant systemic diseases in childhood is found in Table 7. The format of these guidelines did not permit the provision of more details. For more information, please see [9–11].

Table 7. Polyneuropathies in systemic neurological diseases with onset in childhood or adolescence.

Initially Presenting with PNP	+Ataxia	+Spasticity	+Ataxia +Spasticity +EPMS	+Global Developmental Delay	Multisystem Involvement
Metachromatic Leukodystrophy (ARSA)	Vitamin E deficiency (TTPA, MTP, acquired) * Vitamin B12 deficiency * Refsum syndrome (PHYA) * Sensory PNP in Friedreich Ataxia (FXN) EAOH (APTX) SCAR1(SETX) SCA27 (FGF14) AT (ATM) NARP (MTATP6) SCAR23 (PDYN) Microcephaly, seizures, and developmental delay (MCSZ) ARSACS (SACS) SCAN1 (TDP1)	Adrenoleukodystrophy (ABCD1) * Methylmalonic aciduria Vit. B12 deficiency * SPG (4, 9a, 12, 17, 39 ...)	Spastic Aataxia 5 (AFG3L2) LBSL (DARS2) Hypomyelinating leukodystrophy (TUBB4A) Leigh (-like) (SURF1/MFF, SUCLA2)	PDHC (PDHAl) * Krabbe (GALC) * Metachrom. Leukodystrophy (ARSA) * Aicardi-Goutieres syndrome * Global insensitivity to pain (CTLC1) Giant axonal neuropathy (GAN) NBIA2a (PLA2G6) CDG (NGLYl) MCSZ (PNKP) CEDNIK (SNAP29) Ponto-cerebellar hypoplasia (EXOSC3/AMPD2) Infantile Refsum (PEX7)	Mitochondriopathy * multi. acyl CoADH deficiency * Hexosaminidase A/B deficiency (HEXA/HEXB) * Brown–Vialetto-Van Laere (SLC52A2/3) * Peroxisomal 6 (PEX10) ACPHD (ABHD12) PHARC SPOE NBIA (C1901f12) SCAR21 (SCYL1) Familial Dystautonomia (TECPR2) Triple A (AAAS) MEDNIK (AP151) PTRH2 Galaktosialidosis (CTSA)

EAOH: early-onset ataxia, with oculomotor apraxia and hypoalbuminemia; SCAR: spinocerebellar ataxia, recessive; SCA: spinocerebellar ataxia; AT: ataxia teleangiectasia; NARP: neuropathy, ataxia, and retinitis pigmentosa; ARSACS: autosomal recessive spastic ataxia of Charlevoix–Saguenay; SCAN: cerebellar ataxia and sensory-motor axonal neuropathy; SPG: spastic paraplegia; LBSL: leukoencephalopathy with brainstem and spinal cord involvement and lactate elevation; NBIA: neurodegeneration with brain iron accumulation; CDG: carbohydrate deficient glycoprotein disorder; CEDNIK: cerebral dysgenesis, neuropathy, ichthyosis, and palmoplantar keratoderma syndrome; ACPHD: ataxia, combined cerebellar and peripheral, with hearing loss and diabetes mellitus; PHARC: polyneuropathy, hearing loss, ataxia, retinitis pigmentosa, and cataract; MEDNIK: mental retardation, enteropathy, deafness, peripheral neuropathy, ichthyosis, and keratoderma; PTRH: infantile-onset multisystem neurological, endocrine, and pancreatic disease; * **amenable to treatment.**

6. Conclusions

Diseases of the peripheral nerves with highly diverse aetiologies affect children and adolescents as well as adults. The spectrum of their causes in children differs strongly from that of adults. The differential diagnostic approach first requires fundamentally solid anatomical and neurophysiological knowledge and understanding, with thorough analyses of the disease course and family history, the disease's topographic distribution, and the quality of the patient's neurological symptoms. Supplemental examinations such as electrophysiology, laboratory workups, imaging, and CSF diagnostics follow a clinically driven hypothesis. That also applies to molecular genetic diagnostics, which require experience with and a command of the diagnostic algorithms due to the enormous genetic heterogeneity of hereditary neuropathies. These again will be expanded as the potential of broad-based panel or exome diagnostics is realized. To ensure effective and well-targeted therapy, a diagnosis as precise as possible is decisive—not just to alleviate nerve injuries, but also for patients with inflammatory and metabolic/malnutritional neuropathies. The causes of genetic neuropathies should not just be investigated in preparation for genetic counselling. Such knowledge is essential to be able to inform the patient about the disease's probable course and prognosis, and to enable them to participate in present and future clinical trials addressing pathologies and therapies.

Author Contributions: Conceptualization, R.K. and S.R.-S.; methodology, R.K.; software, not applicable; validation, not applicable; formal analysis, not applicable; investigation, not applicable; resources, not applicable; data curation, not applicable; writing—first draft preparation, R.K.; co-ordination of the Delphi process, R.K.; taking part in the Delphi discussion, all authors; writing—review and editing, all authors; visualization, not applicable; supervision, R.K.; project administration, R.K. and R.T.; funding acquisition, R.T. All authors have read and agreed to the published version of the manuscript.

Funding: Translation of the manuscript was funded by the German Speaking Society of Neuropaediatrics.

Institutional Review Board Statement: Not applicable.

Informed Consent Statement: Not applicable.

Data Availability Statement: Not applicable.

Acknowledgments: Publishing Society: Gesellschaft für Neuropädiatrie (R.K., R.T., M.B.). Participating Societies: Deutsche Gesellschaft für Kinder- und Jugendmedizin (R.T.), Deutsche Gesellschaft für Neurologie (B.S.), Deutsche Gesellschaft für Humangenetik (S.R.-S.), Deutsche Gesellschaft für Klinische Neurophysiologie (W.M.-F.), Deutsche Gesellschaft für Neuropathologie und Neuroanatomie (J.W.), Gesellschaft für Pädiatrische Radiologie (N.L., G.H.), Österreichische Gesellschaft für Kinder- und Jugendmedizin (B.P.), Schweizerische Gesellschaft für Neuropädiatrie (G.M.S.), Schweizerische Gesellschaft für Pädiatrie (G.M.S.). We thank Carole Cürten Freiburg for editorial assistance and translation of the manuscript.

Conflicts of Interest: All authors are members of their respective societies. Otherwise, the authors declare no financial or non-financial conflict of interest in developing these guidelines.

References

1. Arbeitsgemeinschaft der Wissenschaftlichen Medizinischen Fachgesellschaften (AWMF)–Ständige Kommission Leitlinien. AWMF-Regelwerk Leitlinien. 1. Auflage. 2012. Available online: http://www.awmf.org/leitlinien/awmf-regelwerk.html (accessed on 20 December 2020).
2. Papazian, O.; Alfonso, I.; Yaylali, I.; Velez, I.; Jayakar, P. Neurophysiological evaluation of children with traumatic radiculopathy, plexopathy, and peripheral neuropathy. *Semin. Pediatr. Neurol.* **2000**, *7*, 26–35. [CrossRef]
3. Blankenburg, M.; Kraemer, N.; Hirschfeld, G.; Krumova, E.K.; Maier, C.; Hechler, T.; Aksu, F.; Magerl, W.; Reinehr, T.; Wiesel, T.; et al. Childhood diabetic neuropathy: Functional impairment and non-invasive screening assessment. *Diabet. Med.* **2012**, *29*, 1425–1432. [CrossRef]
4. Louraki, M.; Karayianni, C.; Kanaka-Gantenbein, C.; Katsalouli, M.; Karavanaki, K. Peripheral neuropathy in children with type 1 diabetes. *Diabet. Metab.* **2012**, *38*, 281–289. [CrossRef]
5. Royden Jones, H., Jr.; De Vivo, D.C.; Darras, B.T. (Eds.) *Neuromuscular Disorders of Infancy, Childhood, and Adolescence*; Butterworth: Amsterdam, The Netherlands, 2003.

6. Williams, S.; Horrocks, I.A.; Ouvrier, R.A.; Gillis, J.; Ryan, M.M. Critical illness polyneuropathy and myopathy in pediatric intensive care: A review. *Pediatr. Crit. Care Med.* **2007**, *8*, 18–22. [CrossRef]
7. Gilchrist, L. Chemotherapy-induced peripheral neuropathy in pediatric cancer patients. *Semin. Pediatr. Neurol.* **2012**, *19*, 9–17. [CrossRef] [PubMed]
8. Rudnik-Schöneborn, S.; Auer-Grumbach, M.; Senderek, J. Charcot-Marie-Tooth disease and hereditary motor neuropathies–update 2020. *Medgen* **2020**, *32*, 207–219.
9. Yiu, E.M.; Ryan, M.M. Demyelinating prenatal and infantile developmental neuropathies. *J. Peripher. Nerv. Syst.* **2012**, *17*, 32–52. [CrossRef]
10. Yiu, E.M.; Ryan, M.M. Genetic axonal neuropathies and neuronopathies of pre-natal and infantile onset. *J. Peripher. Nerv. Syst.* **2012**, *17*, 285–300. [CrossRef] [PubMed]
11. Rossor, A.M.; Carr, A.S.; Devine, H.; Chandrashekar, H.; Pelayo-Negro, A.L.; Pareyson, D.; Shy, M.E.; Scherer, S.S.; Reilly, M.M. Peripheral neuropathy in complex inherited diseases: An approach to diagnosis. *J. Neurol. Neurosurg. Psychiatry* **2017**, *88*, 846–863. [CrossRef] [PubMed]
12. Swoboda, K.J.; Edelbol-Eeg-Oloffson, K.; Harmon, R.L.; Bolton, C.F.; Harper, C.M.; Pitt, M.; Darras, B.T.; Royden Jones, H., Jr. Pediatric Electromyography. In *Neuromuscular Disorders of Infancy, Childhood, and Adolescence*; Royden Jones, H., Jr., De Vivo, D.C., Darras, B.T., Eds.; Butterworth: Amsterdam, The Netherlands, 2003.
13. Pitt, M. Paediatric electromyography in the modern world: A personal view. *Dev. Med. Child Neurol.* **2011**, *53*, 120–124. [CrossRef] [PubMed]
14. Pitt, M.C. Nerve conduction studies and needle EMG in very small children. *Eur. J. Paediatr. Neurol.* **2012**, *16*, 285–291. [CrossRef] [PubMed]
15. Parano, E.; Uncini, A.; De Vivo, D.C.; Lovelace, R.E. Electrophysiologic correlates of peripheral nervous system maturation in infancy and childhood. *J. Child. Neurol.* **1993**, *8*, 336–338. [CrossRef]
16. Plante-Bordeneuve, V. Transthyretin familial amyloid polyneuropathy: An update. *J. Neurol.* **2018**, *265*, 976–983. [CrossRef] [PubMed]
17. Oaklander, A.L.; Nolano, M. Scientific Advances in and Clinical Approaches to Small-Fiber Polyneuropathy: A Review. *JAMA Neurol.* **2019**, *76*, 1240–1251. [CrossRef] [PubMed]
18. Samadi, M.; Kazemi, B.; Golzari Oskoui, S.; Barzegar, M. Assessment of autonomic dysfunction in childhood Guillain-barré syndrome. *J. Cardiovasc. Thorac. Res.* **2013**, *5*, 81–85. [PubMed]
19. Mulkey, S.B.; Glasier, C.M.; El-Nabbout, B.; Walters, W.D.; Ionita, C.; McCarthy, M.H.; Sharp, G.B.; Shbarou, R.M. Nerve root enhancement on spinal MRI in pediatric Guillain-Barre syndrome. *Pediatr. Neurol.* **2010**, *43*, 263–269. [CrossRef]
20. Yikilmaz, A.; Doganay, S.; Gumus, H.; Per, H.; Kumandas, S.; Coskun, A. Magnetic resonance imaging of childhood Guillain-Barre syndrome. *Childs Nerv. Syst.* **2010**, *26*, 1103–1108. [CrossRef]
21. Zuccoli, G.; Panigrahy, A.; Bailey, A.; Fitz, C. Redefining the Guillain-Barre spectrum in children: Neuroimaging findings of cranial nerve involvement. *Am. J. Neuroradiol.* **2011**, *32*, 639–642. [CrossRef] [PubMed]
22. Pham, M.; Bäumer, T.; Bendszus, M. Peripheral nerves and plexus: Imaging by MR-neurography and high-resolution ultrasound. *Curr. Opin. Neurol.* **2014**, *27*, 370–379. [CrossRef]
23. Grimm, A.; Décard, B.F.; Schramm, A.; Pröbstel, A.-K.; Rasenack, M.; Axer, H.; Fuhr, P. Ultrasound and electrophysiologic findings in patients with Guillain–Barré syndrome at disease onset and over a period of six months. *Clin. Neurophysiol.* **2016**, *127*, 1657–1663. [CrossRef] [PubMed]
24. Berciano, J.; Sedano, M.J.; Pelayo-Negro, A.L.; García, A.; Orizaola, P.; Gallardo, E.; Lafarga, M.; Berciano, M.T.; Jacobs, B.C. Proximal nerve lesions in early Guillain–Barré syndrome: Implications for pathogenesis and disease classification. *J. Neurol.* **2017**, *264*, 221–236. [CrossRef] [PubMed]
25. Eggermann, K.; Gess, B.; Häusler, M.; Weis, J.; Hahn, A.; Kurth, I. Hereditary Neuropathies. *Dtsch. Arztebl. Int.* **2018**, *115*, 91–97. [CrossRef] [PubMed]
26. Katona, I.; Weis, J. Diseases of the peripheral nerves. *Handb. Clin. Neurol.* **2018**, *145*, 453–474.
27. Weis, J.; Brandner, S.; Lammens, M.; Sommer, C.; Vallat, J.M. Processing of nerve biopsies: A practical guide for neuropathologists. *Clin. Neuropathol.* **2012**, *31*, 7–23. [CrossRef] [PubMed]
28. Weis, J.; Claeys, K.G.; Roos, A.; Azzedine, H.; Katona, I.; Schröder, J.M.; Senderek, J. Towards a functional pathology of hereditary neuropathies. *Acta Neuropathol.* **2017**, *133*, 493–515. [CrossRef]
29. Nolano, M.; Tozza, S.; Caporaso, G.; Provitera, V. Contribution of Skin Biopsy in Peripheral neuropathies. *Brain Sci.* **2020**, *10*, 989. [CrossRef] [PubMed]
30. Rauer, S.; Kastenbauer, S. Neuroborreliose, S3-Leitlinie 2018. In Deutsche Gesellschaft für Neurologie (Hrsg.). Leitlinien für Diagnostik und Therapie in der Neurologie. Available online: https://dgn.org/leitlinien/ll-030-071-2018-neuroborreliose/ (accessed on 28 June 2021).
31. Malik, V.; Joshi, V.; Green, K.M.; Bruce, I.A. 15 minute consultation: A structured approach to the management of facial paralysis in a child. *Arch. Dis. Child Educ. Pract. Ed.* **2012**, *97*, 82–85. [CrossRef] [PubMed]
32. Ryan, M.M.; Tilton, A.; De Girolami, U.; Darras, B.T.; Jones, H.R., Jr. Paediatric mononeuritis multiplex: A report of three cases and review of the literature. *Neuromuscul. Disord.* **2003**, *13*, 751–756. [CrossRef]

33. Garzoni, L.; Vanoni, F.; Rizzi, M.; Simonetti, G.D.; Goeggel Simonetti, B.; Ramelli, G.P.; Bianchetti, M.G. Nervous system dysfunction in Henoch-Schönlein syndrome: Systematic review of the literature. *Rheumatology* **2009**, *48*, 1524–1529. [CrossRef] [PubMed]
34. Korinthenberg, R.; Trollmann, R.; Felderhoff-Müser, U.; Bernert, G.; Hackenberg, A.; Hufnagel, M.; Pohl, M.; Hahn, G.; Mentzel, H.J.; Sommer, C.; et al. Diagnosis and treatment of Guillain-Barré Syndrome in childhood and adolescence: An evidence- and consensus-based guideline. *Eur. J. Paediatr. Neurol.* **2020**, *25*, 5–16. [CrossRef] [PubMed]
35. Nevo, Y.; Pestronk, A.; Kornberg, A.J.; Connolly, A.M.; Yee, W.C.; Iqbal, I.; Shield, L.K. Childhood chronic inflammatory demyelinating neuropathies: Clinical course and long-term follow-up. *Neurology* **1996**, *47*, 98–102. [CrossRef] [PubMed]
36. McMillan, H.J.; Kang, P.B.; Jones, H.R.; Darras, B.T. Childhood chronic inflammatory demyelinating polyradiculoneuropathy: Combined analysis of a large cohort and eleven published series. *Neuromuscul. Disord.* **2013**, *23*, 103–111. [CrossRef]
37. Korinthenberg, R. Chronic inflammatory demyelinating polyradiculoneuropathy in children and their response to treatment. *Neuropediatrics* **1999**, *30*, 190–196. [CrossRef] [PubMed]
38. Devaux, J.J.; Miura, Y.; Fukami, Y.; Inoue, T.; Manso, C.; Belghazi, M.; Sekiguchi, K.; Kokubun, N.; Ichikawa, H.; Wong, A.H.; et al. Neurofascin-155 IgG4 in chronic inflammatory demyelinating polyneuropathy. *Neurology* **2016**, *86*, 800–807. [CrossRef]
39. Vural, A.; Doppler, K.; Meinl, E. Autoantibodies Against the Node of Ranvier in Seropositive Chronic Inflammatory Demyelinating Polyneuropathy: Diagnostic, Pathogenic, and Therapeutic Relevance. *Front. Immunol.* **2018**, *9*, 1029. [CrossRef]
40. De Simoni, D.; Ricken, G.; Winklehner, M.; Koneczny, I.; Karenfort, M.; Hustedt, U.; Seidel, U.; Abdel-Mannan, O.; Munot, P.; Rinaldi, S.; et al. Antibodies to nodal/paranodal proteins in paediatric immune-mediated neuropathy. *Neurol. Neuroimmunol. Neuroinflamm.* **2020**, *7*, e763. [CrossRef]
41. Fernandez-Garcia, M.A.; Stettner, G.M.; Kinali, M.; Clarke, A.; Fallon, P.; Knirsch, U.; Wraige, E.; Jungbluth, H. Genetic neuropathies presenting with CIDP-like features in childhood. *Neuromuscul. Disord.* **2021**, *31*, 113–122. [CrossRef] [PubMed]
42. Wilmshurst, J.M.; Ouvrier, R. Hereditary peripheral neuropathies of childhood: An overview for clinicians. *Neuromuscul. Disord.* **2011**, *21*, 763–775. [CrossRef] [PubMed]
43. Pipis, M.; Rossor, A.M.; Laura, M.; Reilly, M.M. Next-generation sequencing in Charcot-Marie-Tooth disease: Opportunities and challenges. *Nat. Rev. Neurol.* **2019**, *15*, 644–656. [CrossRef]
44. Baets, J.; Deconinck, T.; De Vriendt, E.; Zimoń, M.; Yperzeele, L.; Van Hoorenbeeck, K.; Peeters, K.; Spiegel, R.; Parman, Y.; Ceulemans, B.; et al. Genetic spectrum of hereditary neuropathies with onset in the first year of life. *Brain* **2011**, *134*, 2664–2676. [CrossRef] [PubMed]
45. Sivera, R.; Sevilla, T.; Vílchez, J.J.; Martínez-Rubio, D.; Chumillas, M.J.; Vázquez, J.F.; Muelas, N.; Bataller, L.; Millán, J.M.; Palau, F.; et al. Charcot-Marie-Tooth disease. Genetic and clinical spectrum in a Spanish clinical series. *Neurology* **2013**, *81*, 1617–1625. [CrossRef] [PubMed]
46. Manganelli, F.; Tozza, S.; Pisciotta, C.; Bellone, E.; Iodice, R.; Nolano, M.; Geroldi, A.; Capponi, S.; Mandich, P.; Santoro, L. Charcot-Marie-Tooth disease: Frequency of genetic subtypes in a Southern Italy population. *J. Peripher. Nerv. Syst.* **2014**, *19*, 292–298. [CrossRef]
47. Rudnik-Schöneborn, S.; Tölle, D.; Senderek, J.; Eggermann, K.; Elbracht, M.; Kornak, U.; von der Hagen, U.; Kirschner, J.; Leube, B.; Müller-Felber, W.; et al. Diagnostic algorithms in Charcot-Marie-Tooth neuropathies: Experiences from a German genetic laboratory on the basis of 1206 index patients. *Clin. Genet.* **2016**, *89*, 34–43. [CrossRef]
48. Liu, X.; Duan, X.; Zhang, Y.; Sun, A.; Fan, D. Molecular analysis and clinical diversity of distal hereditary motor neuropathy. *Eur. J. Neurol.* **2020**, *27*, 1319–1326. [CrossRef]
49. Auer-Grumbach, M. Hereditary sensory and autonomic neuropathies. *Handb. Clin. Neurol.* **2013**, *115*, 893–906. [PubMed]
50. Cox, J.J.; Woods, C.G.; Kurth, I. Peripheral sensory neuropathies–pain loss vs. pain gain. *Medgen* **2020**, *32*, 233–241.

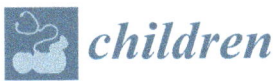

Review

Muscle Ultrasonographic Elastography in Children: Review of the Current Knowledge and Application

Agnieszka Cebula [1,*], Maciej Cebula [2] and Ilona Kopyta [1]

1. Department of Paediatric Neurology, Faculty of Medical Sciences in Katowice, Medical University of Silesia in Katowice, Medykow Str 16, 40-752 Katowice, Poland; ikopyta@sum.edu.pl
2. Department of Radiodiagnostics, Invasive Radiology and Nuclear Medicine, Department of Radiology and Nuclear Medicine, Faculty of Medicine in Katowice, Medical University of Silesia in Katowice, Medykow Str 14, 40-752 Katowice, Poland; mcebula@sum.edu.pl
* Correspondence: d200907@365.sum.edu.pl; Fax: +48-322071546

Abstract: Ultrasonographic elastography is a relatively new imaging modality for the qualitative and quantitative assessments of tissue elasticity. While it has steadily gained use in adult clinical practice, including for liver diseases, breast cancer, thyroid pathologies, and muscle and tendon diseases, data on its paediatric application is still limited. Moreover, diagnosis of muscular diseases in children remains challenging. The gold standard methods, namely biopsy, electroneurography, and electromyography, are often limited owing to their invasive characteristics, possible contraindications, complications, and need for good cooperation, that is, a patient's ability to perform certain tasks during the examination while withstanding discomfort, which is a significant problem especially in younger or uncooperative children. Genetic testing, which has broad diagnostic possibilities, often entails a high cost, which limits its application. Thus, a non-invasive, objective, repeatable, and accessible tool is needed to aid in both the diagnosis and monitoring of muscle pathologies. We believe that elastography may prove to be such a method. The aim of this review was to present the current knowledge on the use of muscle elastography in the paediatric population and information on the limitations of elastography in relation to examination protocols and factors for consideration in everyday practice and future studies.

Keywords: ultrasonographic elastography; neuromuscular disease; muscle; children

1. Introduction

The diagnosis and monitoring of neuromuscular diseases remain a challenge despite the emerging role of genetic testing in this field. Vital limitations in diagnosis and monitoring are particularly relevant in the paediatric group owing to the high costs of genetic tests and invasiveness of gold standard tests (electromyography (EMG), electroneurography (ENG), and biopsy). Both ENG and EMG require good patient compliance (ability to simultaneously withstand discomfort and relax or contract muscles on demand), may lead to complications like most invasive procedures, and are often limited by the need to ensure patient safety and health-related contraindications. Thus, a new, non-invasive, affordable, and objective test is urgently needed. We believe that elastography may prove to be such a tool in the future, as it has already been applied in hepatological, endocrinal, and oncological diagnostics [1,2]. Although far more studies on muscle elastography have been conducted in the adult population than in children, results from the former cannot be simply applied to the latter. Thus, the aim of this study was to present existing elastography modalities, their limitations, and applications in paediatric muscle-related disorders.

Technical Aspects of Elastography

Elastography is an assessment method based on the elastic properties of soft tissues. A few modalities based on magnetic resonance (MR) and ultrasonography (US) already

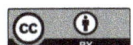

exist. However, we limited the present study to US modalities, as they are easier to access in everyday clinical work, provide real-time metrics for most cases, and are less costly. Studies that compared elastography from MR and different US methods in children are scarce, and their results remain inconsistent [3–5].

The main US elastographic modalities are strain elastography (SE), acoustic radiation force impulse (ARFI), transient elastography (TE), and shear wave elastography (SWE). In general, the main distinctive differences are the method of stress application, detection of tissue deformation, and characteristics of gained data (qualitative vs. quantitative). A simplified classification of elastographic methods is presented on Figure 1. One of the most important impediments in elastographic research analysis is provider-dependant varieties, subdivision of modalities, and inconsistency in nomenclature.

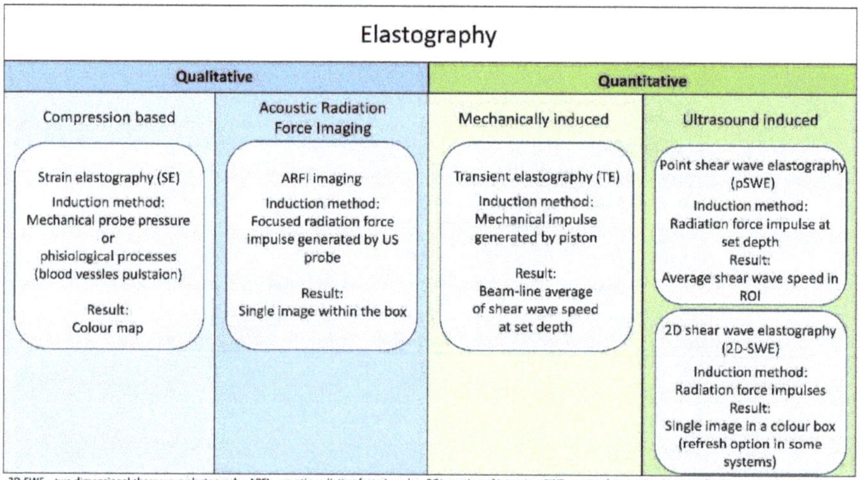

Elastography			
Qualitative		**Quantitative**	
Compression based	Acoustic Radiation Force Imaging	Mechanically induced	Ultrasound induced
Strain elastography (SE) Induction method: Mechanical probe pressure or phisiological processes (blood vessels pulstaion) Result: Colour map	ARFI imaging Induction method: Focused radiation force impulse generated by US probe Result: Single image within the box	Transient elastography (TE) Induction method: Mechanical impulse generated by piston Result: Beam-line average of shear wave speed at set depth	Point shear wave elastography (pSWE) Induction method: Radiation force impulse at set depth Result: Average shear wave speed in ROI
			2D shear wave elastography (2D-SWE) Induction method: Radiation force impulses Result: Single image in a colour box (refresh option in some systems)

2D-SWE – two dimensional shear wave elastography, ARFI – acustic radiation force impulse, ROI – region of interest, pSWE – point shear wave elastography, SE – strain elastography, TE – transient elastography, US – ultrasound.

Figure 1. Simplified division of elastographic methods.

SE is currently widely available, as it is offered by most leading manufacturers of US devices. The qualitative measurement is based on the amount of strain that is mechanically induced by either the mechanical pressure of the US probe or physiological processes such as blood vessel pulsation. The effect is presented as a colour map, with some vendors offering software for semi-quantitative analysis such as strain ratio (SR) calculation. Among the SE methods, a Hitachi-patented real-time elastography device has gained the most interest. It implements the extended combined autocorrelation method, an algorithm that correlates in both axial and lateral directions and produces an elasticity image in real time. Despite the implementation of various quality-control systems, the method is still heavily operator-dependant [1,6].

ARFI imaging is a Siemens-patented qualitative method based on the focused radiation force impulse produced by the US probe, whose displacement is evaluated at the set depth. The results are shown as a single image within the box. The attainability with systems by a single manufacturer is a valid availability limitation [1].

TE is the first quantitative method designed by Echosens for the evaluation of liver fibrosis and steatosis. A specifically designed piston induces a mechanical impulse, and US is used for beam-line average measurement of the resulting shear wave speed. Owing to its design, this method has not played a major role in muscular evaluation [1].

SWE is a group of methods that can be roughly divided into point and two-dimensional (2-D) SWEs, with further subdivision according to the method of force application. From a practical point of view, all these methods measure shear wave speed and offer quantitative results expressed in meters per second, which are subsequently converted to kilopascals by using the Young modulus. One of the main limitations is the assumption of homogeneity of the wave propagation medium, which is usually not the case with muscles. Other limitations include the manufacturer-dependent method of induction and calculation of shear wave speed, which make a direct comparison of vendor results impossible [1,7,8]. SWE and ARFI may also be affected by the depth of examined tissues [7,9–11]. As in the paediatric population, tight muscle thickness was reported to be up to 45 mm. Thus, SWE might have a broader application in this age group [12]. In general the most commonly used devices are Aixplorer (Supersonic Imagine, Aix-en-Provence, France), which supports 2-D SWE, and Acuson (S2000/S3000; Siemens, Washington, DC, USA), which generates ARFI [13].

2. Materials and Methods

A thorough literature search on the PubMed database was performed using the MeSH terms "elasticity imaging techniques/methods", "child", and "muscle", and search words with the search operator AND ("elastography", "child", "muscle", and "children"). After the initial search of manuscripts from 2012 to 2020, 1329 studies were found. We limited the number of studies to 58 by manually checking articles and their abstracts. In addition, their bibliographies were analysed and checked. Studies that did not involve children, those that analysed only different muscular tissues (including studies on tendons only), those that had only the abstract available, duplicate articles, short reviews of the general use of elastography, those that involved only MR elastography, and those that were in languages other either Polish or English were excluded. Finally, 35 articles were included in this study. A summary of the process is presented in Figure 2.

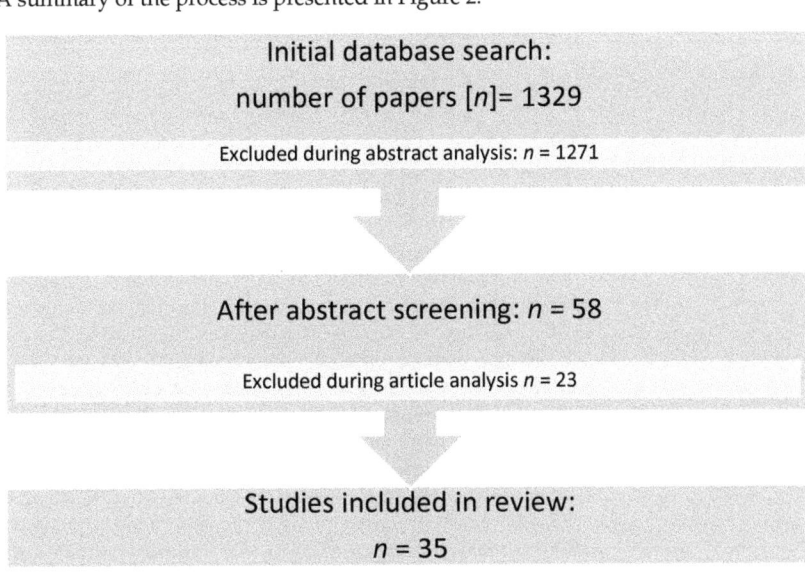

Figure 2. Flow diagram of the literature search.

The results presented were divided into two parts as follows: one is the technical and demographic aspects that influence the results, and the other is current knowledge on muscle elastography results in different clinical problems in children.

3. Factors Influencing Elastography

The following subparagraphs focus on factors affecting the elastography results that are not connected to the patient's disease. The sex, age, anthropometry, muscle stretching, tissue compression and operator-related reliability are discussed in turns.

3.1. Differences Related to Patient Sex

While multiple factors may influence muscular status, data regarding the association between patient sex and elastography results are too limited to form a clear conclusion. However, few studies have observed no sex-related differences between modalities in small children.

Brandenburg et al. found no significant sex-related difference in a study of SWE of the gastrocnemius muscle (GCM) in 20 healthy children aged 2 to 12 years. All the patients were in their prepubertal age [14]. No significant difference in ARFI was found in a study in 12 children with cerebral palsy (CP) aged 6 to 14 years and a study of SWE of the GCM in 86 patients from different age groups [15,16]. The latter involved 27 children (6–12 years) and 59 adults, but the authors did not assess the association of sex to muscles stiffness separately for the different age groups [15].

On the other hand, Koppenhaver et al. evaluated 130 adult patients to study factors that affect lumbar muscle stiffness on SWE. In this study, significant differences were found between men and women in all the muscles evaluated, with larger shear modules in the men. The authors estimated that the values for the male group were approximately 20% higher than those for the female group across all the examined lower back muscles in both the relaxed and contracted states [16]. Significant sex-related differences in ARFI and SWE findings were also described in other studies in adult populations [9,17,18]. One study of 42 healthy children found that there was significant difference between male and female's rectus femoris muscle but only at rest [19].

This sex-related disparity in elastography results between age groups and studies has raised the question of whether the observed changes might be dependent on maturity and the location and type of the examined muscles. More data are needed to clarify this.

3.2. Age-Related Differences

Increase in muscle stiffness with age was clearly described in some adult studies [9,17]. A similar tendency was observed in paediatric studies, with some minor deviations [14,15,20–22].

Liu et al. evaluated the GCMs of 86 healthy volunteers, divided into three age groups (paediatric: <16 years, middle-aged: 30–40 years, and old: >55 years). While no statistically significant differences were found in the plantar flexion (PF) and neutral positions of the feet, a significant increase in muscle stiffness in dorsiflexion (at all angles of the ankle from $10°$ to $30°$) was observed with age [15]. In a study by Wenz et al. that compared the SE results of the upper and lower limb muscles in young adults (22 patients, aged 20–30 years) and children (21 patients, aged 2–12 years), significant differences were found between the two groups [20]. Brandenburg et al. assessed muscle changes in 20 children (aged 2–12 years) and found that muscle stiffness increased with age but it did not reach statistical significance [14].

An interesting trend was described in a study of Achilles tendons in Turkish paediatric populations with and without CP. A significant difference in age was found, but while the SR increased with age in the CP group ($p < 0.001$), it showed an inverse correlation with age in the healthy group ($p = 0.038$). The authors concluded that changes in muscle stiffness not only occur due to ageing but also may show specific patterns of ageing in different diseases [22]. In a study in patients with Duchenne muscular dystrophy (DMD) aged 5 to 24 years, results were incoherent in that while a statistical correlation was found between age and GCM stiffness in the DMD group, no correlation was found in the healthy group or for other muscles in the DMD group [21].

3.3. Differences Related to Anthropometry and Anisotropy

No relationship was found between muscle stiffness and calf circumference in healthy subjects. A tendency for decreasing muscle stiffness in relation to increasing BMI was observed but did not reach statistical significance. Range of movement and foot dominance did not influence muscle stiffness [14]. Another study on children population presented incoherent results: while higher BMI was related with decrease of biceps brachii long elasticity immediately after exercise, but none at rest, for rectus femoris muscle it was the other way around. The authors found significant rise of elasticity with higher BMI but only at rest and not following exercise [19]. In the adult population in the study of Koppenhaver et al., a clear association was found between BMI, self-assessed activity level, and SWE results [16].

Gennison et al. studied the effect of a muscle's anisotropy, i.e., changes in mechanical properties along with the direction of measurement [23]. The longitudinal direction is recognized as the most relevant, as the muscle mechanical properties change with its lengthening and shortening [21,24]. The impact of the muscle anisotropy is still a subject of intensive research, with almost a hundred papers published annually. Yet, probably due to mentioned study results–authors of cited papers used longitudinal direction in their studies.

3.4. Passive Muscle Stretching Influences Study Results

Few studies focused on muscle stretching-related changes in muscle elasticity. Most of these studies assessed GCM changes as the effects of ankle joint dorsiflexion (DF), PF, and neutral position. Even though clear methodological differences (regarding the exact ankle angle measured, knee flexion, the study protocol used, and the tools used to ensure planned feet position) were present, the results were coherent; passive stiffness increased as a result of increased DF angle [14,15,25]. In a study of SWE of the anterior tibialis (AT) muscle and GCM in hemiplegic patients, Lee et al. confirmed that ankle angle had significant effects on both muscles. The study demonstrated a quadratic relationship between ankle angle and SW speed [26]. In a study by Brandenburg et al., muscle stiffness on SWE at 10° dorsiflexion was 4 times higher than at 20° PF [14]. Lacourpaille et al. proved that while muscle stiffness differed between patients with DMD and their healthy peers in 5 of 6 examined muscles during muscle stretching, this difference was present in only 3 muscles when no stretching was applied [21]. Thus, we may conclude that muscle stretching substantially changes muscle stiffness, especially in neuromuscular diseases, and not taking it into consideration may lead to errors in the study results and diagnosis.

Caliskan et al. focused on different aspects of muscle stretching. They studied whether the duration of passive muscle stretching affected muscle elasticity on SWE. Twenty male athletes aged 12 to 16 years were recruited. SWE was performed before and after 2 min (group 1) and 5 min (group 2) of passive stretching. While in the first group, no significant differences in pre-stretching results were found, significant reduction in muscle stiffness was observed in group 2 after 5 min. Even though the study population was small and limited to one sex, apart from the practical conclusions for sport medicine and physiotherapy, this study showed that the elastography examination protocol should carefully consider passive muscle stretching [25].

3.5. Exercise and Effort's Effect on Muscle Elasticity

Apart from mentioned above effect of stretching, effort and exercise lead to changes seen in elastography on their own. In a study of 40 paediatric patients, Berko et al. proved that results of strain elastography before and immediately after leading to fatigue exercise significantly differed. The post-exercise elasticity of both biceps brachii long and rectus femoris muscle was lower [19]. This effect must be taken into account while planning clinical use of muscle elastography.

3.6. Influence of Tissue Compression on Elastography

As muscle tissue reacts to compression and passive elongation, with possible exacerbation of the reaction in some neuromuscular diseases, the question of whether force applied by the US probe changes the elastography results remains valid. In most of the studies included in this analysis, researchers decided to minimise the effect by either performing the study with as little compression as possible or reducing the distortion of the subcutaneous soft tissue with the use of a generous amount of US gel [4,14,18,27,28]. The latter solution might have an important limitation as seen in a study in 23 adult patients by Alfuraih et al. The authors compared SWEs of the vastus lateralis muscle with minimal pressure applied to the skin and with "standoff gel" applied at a minimum thickness of 5 mm. While no significant changes in mean shear wave speed was found between the groups, the reliability quantified by intraclass correlation coefficient (ICC) decreased from near-perfect agreement (ICC = 0.83) to the margin of substantial agreement (ICC = 0.62) in the gel method [7]. Further studies on the compression effect of the probe on elastography results are needed.

3.7. Operator-Related Reliability

A few studies assessed inter- and intra-operator reliability as moderate to excellent regardless of the muscle evaluated and modalities used (ICC, from >0.6 to >0.9) [24,29–31] A. While no relationship between BMI and elastography results in children were described by Linek et al., they found that the thickness of fat tissue above the lateral abdominal muscles influenced the reliability of the results of their study. Thinner fat layers (<5 mm on average) had positive influences on inter-rater reliability. In addition, the side of the examined muscle carried consequences as well. Worse inter- and intra-operator reliability results were observed when the examined muscle was on the patient's side opposite to the examiner. This again may be the result of the different pressures applied by the probe and thus again raises the question on methodology [29].

4. Elastography in Different Muscle Disorders

The following subparagraphs focus on the elastography results in relation to the patient's muscles disease. The muscular dystrophies, other myopathies, cerebral palsy and its treatment are discussed in turns.

4.1. Muscle Elastography in Muscular Dystrophies

As research on treatment strategies for myopathies has been progressing over the recent years, the need for treatment monitoring tools is also increasing. Few studies have presented differences between healthy peers and patients with DMD. Lacourpaille, Lilian, et al. compared results from different muscles in a healthy group (n = 13) and a DMD group (n = 14) of patients aged 5–24 years. While significant differences in muscle stiffness were found in the AT, GCM, vastus lateralis, biceps, and triceps brachii, the difference in muscle stiffness of the abductor digiti brevis minimi did not reach statistical significance. The highest difference was observed in the vastus lateralis, with the stiffness 134% higher in the DMD group [21]. Pichiecchio et al. compared the SWE and MRI results of the lower limb muscles (GCM, AT, rectus femoris, vastus lateralis and medialis, adductor magnus, and gluteus maximus) from 5 children with DMD with those from their age-matched healthy peers. Moderately higher muscle stiffness values were found in the DMD group. However, no significant correlation was found between the SWE and MRI results for fat replacement and muscle oedema on T1 and short inversion-time inversion-recovery (STIR) images. Although the study was limited by both the small number of participants and inclusion of a patient with a milder clinical presentation and mutation associated with Becker dystrophy, it presented the question of whether MRI and SWE analyse overlapping or different aspects of muscle diseases and if they can be used interchangeably. In addition, the patient with a clinical presentation of Becker dystrophy showed interesting results in that the changes in the SWE values were not accompanied by fat or STIR changes on MRI and clinical abnormalities in the patient examinations, which possibly preceded the latter [4]. The hypothesis that elastography might be useful as a screening tool thus remains to be proven.

Furthermore, by analysing changes in SWE results from patients with DMD over 12 months, Lacourpaille proved that elastography is a good candidate monitoring tool. They compared resting shear modules from the AT, GCM, biceps and triceps brachii, and abductor digiti minimi muscles in 10 children with genetically confirmed DMD and 9 age-matched healthy peers. While no significant changes over time were found in the control group, the DMD group showed significant increases in the AT (75.1% ± 93.5%, $p = 0.043$), GCM (144.8% ± 180.6%, $p = 0.050$), and triceps brachii (35.5% ± 32.2%, $p = 0.005$). The biceps brachii and abductor digiti minimi muscle changes did not reach statistical significance [32].

4.2. Other Myopathies

Berko et al. designed a study to evaluate the usefulness and efficacy of SE for juvenile idiopathic inflammatory myopathies (JIIMs) and compared them with those of MRI. The authors recruited 18 patients aged 3 to 19 years, assessed the clinical activity of the disease, and performed both MRI of the pelvic region and thighs and strain elastography of the quadriceps muscles. The results were not favourable for SE. While the MRI results were related to disease activity ($p = 0.012$), the elastography results showed no association with either the MRI results or disease activity. Also no relationship was found between elastography and disease duration; thus, the results cannot be simply explained by the shorter disease time in the adults [5]. The question remains as to whether qualitative and less operator-dependent elastographic modalities would provide better results, as JIIMs are expected to affect muscle elasticity.

By contrast, Song et al. examined the SEs of patients with inflammatory myopathies, regardless of age. They proved that the affected muscles had higher strain rates and that SR correlated with the pathological scores of the biopsy samples [12]. However, as only one of the 17 patients was a child (an 11-year-old girl with juvenile dermatomyositis) and her SR was lower than those of the other participants, no conclusion for the paediatric population may be given from this study. This also implies the possibility that age influences elastography results.

4.3. Cerebral Palsy

CP is one of the most common disorders associated with secondary muscle changes in the paediatric population. Owing to the large number of patients, the patterns of changes found in affected muscles, and the treatments aimed at decreasing muscle spasticity, only a few studies on elastography in CP already exist.

Few studies focused on assessing the differences between muscles affected and those not affected by CP. Kwon at al compared strain and ARFI results from the GCM and soleus muscle in 15 patients with CP and 13 healthy peers, all aged <13 years. The GCM had greater muscle stiffness on SE and higher ARFI velocity in the CP group. While the soleus muscle had higher values on SE, its shear wave velocity was similar in both the CP and healthy groups. The SR (ratio of the GCM to the soleus muscle) was significantly higher in the CP group than in the healthy group. The authors concluded that the GCM had greater involvement in the motor deficits in CP [33]. In another study, Lee at al., based on a group of 7 children with hemiplegic CP and 1 post-stroke paediatric patient with similar clinical presentations, proved that the AT and GCM had significantly different SW speeds between the less and more affected sides. Patients with Gross Motor Function Classification System levels I and II, indicating no gross motor deficits, were compared. In the neutral joint position, the mean SW speed was 20% higher for the AT on the more affected side (3.86 m/s vs. 3.22 m/s, $p = 0.03$) and 14% higher for the GCM (5.04 m/s vs. 4/46 m/s, $p = 0.024$) [26]. Ozturk et al. compared Achilles tendon stiffness between CP patients (72 children, CP group) and their healthy peers (83 children, control group). The control group had lower SR than the CP group (1.7 ± 0.1 vs. 4.1 ± 0.8, $p < 0.001$) [22]. On the basis of the SWEs of the soleus muscle in 21 children with CP and 21 healthy peers, Vola et al. proved that muscle elasticity differed significantly between the hemiplegic and healthy patients. Higher Young modulus values were found in the CP group than in the healthy group (8.1 ± 2.3 kPa vs. 4.8 ± 1.7 kPa, $p < 0.001$) [34]. Similar results were presented for ARFI by Bilgici et al. In their study in 17 children with CP and 25 healthy peers, they compared GCM elasticity and modified Ashworth scale (MAS) scores. The mean shear wave velocity was 3.17 ± 0.81 m/s in the CP group and 1.45 ± 0.25 m/s in the control group ($p < 0.001$) [35]. A recent study by Lallemant-Dudek et al. compared SWE results of GCM and biceps brachii long. Paper has some important limitations as the control group included patients with scoliosis while no information on possible muscle disease was given and in addition some of the patients from CP did receive botulin toxin (BoNT-A) treatment. Yet authors found that while there was no difference between groups when muscle was at rest, CP involved muscles differed from both–control group and uninvolved muscles in CP patients [36]. In other study, Mansouri et al. confirmed the relationship of the elastography results of the anterior tibialis muscle and GCM with gait abnormalities (step time and walking speed) [28]. Some studies confirmed that muscle stiffness assessed using elastography is related with clinical presentations assessed using MAS score [34,35]. While in others no such correlation was found [36].

To test the hypothesis that hyperactivity and spasticity of the hip abductors and flexors result in the hip displacement in CP, Doruk Analan et al. analysed the correlation between the Reimers hip migration index and the elasticity of the mentioned muscles on SWE. No significant correlation was found [37].

4.4. CP Treatment Evaluation Using Elastography

The use of elastography in monitoring botulin toxin A (BoNT-A) treatment in patients with CP is gaining attention. Studies that showed changes in muscle stiffness after BoNT-A administration into GCMs in children are presented in Table 1. In addition, some authors presented clear associations between post-BoNT-A changes in elastography result and clinical scale scores for spasticity (MAS and modified Tardieu scale [MTS]) [27,35,38]. By assessing post-BoNT-A elasticity changes of the anterior tibialis in addition to those of the gastrocnemius, Dag et al. proved that botulin treatment affects not only the muscle where BoNT-A was administrated but also the overall patient gait and related muscles. In some patients, paradoxical increases in shear wave speed were observed regardless of changes in MAS score, probably due to abnormal collagen content, injection failure, wrong injection site, insufficient dose, and so forth. In such cases, measurement of changes between the pre- and post-elastography values combined with US might prove to be a useful tool for further decision making regarding eventual treatment withdrawal [39]. In addition to mentioned studies that focused on the treatment effects at one month post BoNT-A administration, in a study in 9 children aged 2 to 9 years, Brandenburg et al. quantified the duration of treatment effect. They set three study visits up to 1 month before and 1 and 3 months after injection. While near-significant differences were found between the pre-BoNT-A administration and first post-treatment control, no significant difference was found between the pre- and 3-month post-BoNT-A values. The most significant difference was found between the 1- and 3-month post-BoNT-A values. Thus, the authors showed that the BoNT-A effect on muscle stiffness on SWE lasted <3 months post injection. SWE proved to be a reliable tool for individualised monitoring and planning of botulin treatment in patients with CP [40]. We can then conclude that elastography might be useful in the most effective and patient-tailored BoNT-A therapy by guiding administration planning, determining the treatment prognosis, allowing for objective treatment assessment (e.g., comparison between elastography-based MAS and MTS scores less subjectively and isolated muscle assessment rather than combined assessment of muscles, joints, tendons, surrounding tissues, and excitability changes), and guiding the choice of the best time interval between doses.

Table 1. Studies on the relationship between elastography and BoNT-A treatment in cerebral palsy.

Study	Method	Population	Muscle Assessed	Before BoNT-A	1 Month after BoNT-A	p Value
Ceyhan Bilgici et al., 2018 [39]	ARFI	n = 12 (6♀) 8.58 ± 2.48 yo	Gastrocnemius	SWS: 3.20 ± 0.14 m/s	SWS: 2.45 ± 0.21 m/s	<0.01
Park and Kwon, 2012 [38]	SE	n = 17 (7♀) 4.75 ± 1.83 yo	Medial gastrocnemius	RTS score: 3.4	RTS score: 1.5	<0.05
Dağ et al., 2020 [27]	SWE	n = 24 (10♀) 2–11 yo	Lateral gastrocnemius	Stiffness: 45.9 ± 6.5 kPa	Stiffness: 25.0 ± 5.7 kPa	<0.01
			Anterior tibialis	Stiffness: 36.9 ± 7.9 kPa	Stiffness: 28.4 ± 5.2 kPa	<0.01
Brandenburg et al., 2018 [40]	SWE	n = 9 (4♀) 2–9 yo	Lateral gastrocnemius	0° PF	1 month vs. 3 months after BoNT-A*	0.02
				10° PF		0.03

ARFI, acoustic radiation force impulse; BoNT-A*, botulin toxin A; PF, plantar flexion; RTS, real-time sonoelastography; SE, strain elastography; SWE, shear wave elastography; SWS, shear wave speed; yo, years old.

5. Muscle Elastography in Other Diseases

The following subparagraphs focus on the elastography results in relation to other diseases influencing muscle tissue. The chronic kidney diseases, gluteus muscle contracture, torticollis, Osgood-Schlatter disease, elbow injuries, musculoskeletal tumours are be discussed in turns.

5.1. Chronic Kidney Diseases

In their study, Bekci et al. assessed the possible use of ARFI in screening for muscle changes in chronic kidney diseases (CKDs). The reason for the muscle function loss in CKD is still not fully elucidated, but factors such as disease-related myopathy, muscle loss, and abnormal fat deposition are considered possible causes. The study population consisted of children aged 6 to 17 years, including 23 patients with CKD (11 girls) and 22 healthy peers (11 girls). The authors performed an elastographic evaluation of the elasticity of the rectus femoris muscle and handheld dynamometry (HHD) for evaluation of the maximal isometric strength of the knee extensors. The results showed that both muscle strength and elasticity were significantly decreased in the CKD group compared with the healthy volunteers. Whereas HHD has limited reliability, the authors concluded that elastographic techniques might prove feasible, affordable, and objective tools for treatment planning, monitoring, and screening for muscle changes [35].

5.2. Gluteus Muscle Contracture

Gluteus muscle contracture is a clinical syndrome most often found in the age group of 6–18 years, in relation to the above-mentioned pathological muscle changes, and is characterised by abnormal gait and hip movement limitations (mainly flexion and adduction). Diagnosis is often delayed and thus affects the prognosis, which is closely related to early treatment (surgery being the gold standard). In a small group of three patients, Guo et al. proved that measurement of muscle stiffness using SWE might be useful in the diagnosis. They speculated that SWE results may be related to the severity of the syndrome, making elastography a potentially useful tool for the assessment needed for treatment and prognosis [41].

5.3. Torticollis

Lee at al performed strain elastography of the sternocleidomastoid muscle and compared the results between infants with congenital torticollis and their healthy peers. The torticollis group had significantly lower muscle elasticity values [31]. The authors concluded that elastography may be a useful tool for monitoring and diagnosing torticollis especially in cases with subtle changes.

5.4. Osgood-Schlatter Disease

On the basis of real-time tissue elastography results of the rectus femoris muscles in 37 teenage male athletes, Enomoto et al. rejected the hypothesis that one of the factors that lead to Osgood-Schlatter disease is higher-than-normal muscle stiffness. No significant difference in quadriceps muscle stiffness was found between the OGD and healthy groups [2].

5.5. Elbow Injuries Related to Sports

In a study based on strain elastography results of the upper limb muscles in 197 baseball players aged 9 to 15 years, Saito et al. focused on addressing the question as to whether elbow injuries are related to pronator teres muscle (PTM) stiffness. The muscle group functions as a dynamic stabiliser against elbow valgus force. According to US results, the participants were divided into three groups, namely those with medial epicondylar fragmentation in the throwing arm, those with osteochondritis dissecans (OCD) of the humoral capitellum, and healthy peers. The elasticity of the pronator teres muscle was significantly higher in both injury groups than in the healthy group. In addition, the authors found that while only the muscle spasticity of the throwing arm was significantly higher in the OCD group, the PTMs on both sides were affected in the medial elbow injury group. The authors concluded that this may prove that medial elbow injury might be the result of muscle changes, not the other way around; thus, screening for muscle stiffness changes might help prevent the injury. Moreover, by comparing the strain results between the range of movement of the upper limb and those of the elbow and arm joints (with significant differences only for external rotation of the glenohumeral joint), the authors remarked that the changes in muscle spasticity observed on elastography might precede those observed in clinical examinations [30].

5.6. Oncology: Musculoskeletal Tumours

Timely detection and diagnosis of suspicious lesions are often the factors that lead to better treatment efficacy. However, the heterogeneity of pathological masses challenges all available techniques. Li et al. evaluated the usefulness of real-time 2-D SWE in distinguishing between benign and malignant musculoskeletal lesions by examining 115 tumours in 92 children and adults. Both quantitative (minimum, maximum, and mean elasticity in kilopascals) and qualitative (colour map sale) elastography results were analysed in comparison with the histopathological evaluation results. All the parameters were significantly different between the benign and malignant tumours ($p < 0.05$). By performing a multivariate regression analysis, the mean elasticity values were found to have strongest independent prediction for malignancy, with 71.4% accuracy, 66.7% sensitivity, and 85% specificity. In the same study, the authors also compared the diagnostic efficacy of US with those of both qualitative and quantitative SWEs. They found no significant differences in diagnostic efficacy, which was considered moderate for all the techniques. Assessment of lesion stiffness proved to be an important addition in morphological evaluations. One of the important limitation of this study was the exclusion of tumours exceeding the maximal region of interest of 4×6.5 cm [42].

6. Study Limitations and Conclusions

Since most existing studies have different study protocols in relation to the different positions of the analysed limb/muscles, which affected the acquired measurements; the stretching protocol; the non-homogenous groups with regard to age and sex; and the lack of standardisation of the pressure generated by the transducers on the patients' skin and muscles, the results of the studies included in our analysis were not comparable in most aspects.

Further studies are needed to develop normative values for different age groups that account for developmental changes, to characterise the influences of sex on the normative values, to standardise the test protocol, and to assess whether skin and tissue compression significantly changes measured values. Moreover, further investigation into the probe position on muscles (perpendicular and distal/proximal positions), the influence of body temperature, muscle stretching, different muscles, and the relationships of stiffness values to clinical characteristics (e.g., hypotonia) and other diagnostic tools are needed. Nevertheless, application of this imaging modality is a promising direction for the diagnosis and monitoring of muscular diseases. Development of unified examination protocols and further objectification of muscle elastography may be an important step for better understanding, recognition, and monitoring of the different muscle pathologies in specific, non-easily cooperating group of small patients.

Author Contributions: Conceptualization, A.C. and M.C.; methodology, A.C.; software, M.C.; validation, A.C., M.C. and I.K.; formal analysis, I.K.; investigation, A.C.; resources, M.C.; writing—original draft preparation, A.C., M.C.; writing—review and editing, A.C., M.C., I.K.; visualization, A.C., M.C.; supervision, I.K.; project administration, M.C.; funding acquisition, M.C. All authors have read and agreed to the published version of the manuscript.

Funding: This research received no external funding.

Institutional Review Board Statement: Not applicable.

Informed Consent Statement: Not applicable.

Conflicts of Interest: The authors declare no conflict of interest.

References

1. Dietrich, C.; Bamber, J.; Berzigotti, A.; Bota, S.; Cantisani, V.; Castera, L.; Cosgrove, D.; Ferraioli, G.; Friedrich-Rust, M.; Gilja, O.H.; et al. EFSUMB Guidelines and Recommendations on the Clinical Use of Liver Ultrasound Elastography, Update 2017 (Long Version). *Ultraschall Med.* **2017**, *38*, e16–e47. [CrossRef]
2. Enomoto, S.; Tsushima, A.; Oda, T.; Kaga, M. The passive mechanical properties of muscles and tendons in children affected by Osgood-Schlatter disease. *J. Pediatr. Orthop.* **2020**, *40*, e243–e247. [CrossRef] [PubMed]
3. Debernard, L.; Robert, L.; Charleux, F.; Bensamoun, S.F. A possible clinical tool to depict muscle elasticity mapping using magnetic resonance elastography. *Muscle Nerve* **2013**, *47*, 903–908. [CrossRef]
4. Pichiecchio, A.; Alessandrino, F.; Bortolotto, C.; Cerica, A.; Rosti, C.; Raciti, M.V.; Rossi, M.; Berardinelli, A.; Baranello, G.; Bastianello, S.; et al. Muscle ultrasound elastography and MRI in preschool children with Duchenne muscular dystrophy. *Neuromuscul. Disord.* **2018**, *28*, 476–483. [CrossRef]
5. Berko, N.S.; Hay, A.; Sterba, Y.; Wahezi, D.; Levin, T.L. Efficacy of ultrasound elastography in detecting active myositis in children: Can it replace MRI? *Pediatr. Radiol.* **2015**, *45*, 1522–1528. [CrossRef]
6. Ewertsen, C.; Carlsen, J.F.; Christiansen, I.R.; Jensen, J.A.; Nielsen, M.B. Evaluation of healthy muscle tissue by strain and shear wave elastography—Dependency on depth and ROI position in relation to underlying bone. *Ultrasonics* **2016**, *71*, 127–133. [CrossRef]
7. Alfuraih, A.M.; O'Connor, P.; Hensor, E.; Tan, A.L.; Emery, P.; Wakefield, R.J. The effect of unit, depth, and probe load on the reliability of muscle shear wave elastography: Variables affecting reliability of SWE. *J. Clin. Ultrasound* **2018**, *46*, 108–115. [CrossRef] [PubMed]
8. Gilligan, L.A.; Trout, A.T.; Bennett, P.; Dillman, J.R. Repeatability and agreement of shear wave speed measurements in phantoms and human livers across 6 Ultrasound 2-Dimensional shear wave elastography systems. *Investig. Radiol.* **2020**, *55*, 191–199. [CrossRef]
9. Heizelmann, A.; Tasdemir, S.; Schmidberger, J.; Gräter, T.; Kratzer, W.; Grüner, B. Measurements of the trapezius and erector spinae muscles using virtual touch imaging quantification ultrasound-Elastography: A cross section study. *BMC Musculoskelet. Disord.* **2017**, *18*, 370. [CrossRef]
10. Wang, X.; Hu, Y.; Zhu, J.; Gao, J.; Chen, S.; Liu, F.; Li, W.; Liu, Y.; Ariun, B. Effect of acquisition depth and precompression from probe and couplant on shear wave elastography in soft tissue: An in vitro and in vivo study. *Quant. Imaging Med. Surg.* **2020**, *10*, 754–765. [CrossRef] [PubMed]
11. Shin, H.J.; Kim, M.J.; Kim, H.Y.; Roh, Y.H.; Lee, M.J. Comparison of shear wave velocities on ultrasound elastography between different machines, transducers, and acquisition depths: A phantom study. *Eur. Radiol.* **2016**, *26*, 3361–3367. [CrossRef]
12. Song, Y.; Lee, S.; Yoo, D.H.; Jang, K.S.; Bae, J. Strain sonoelastography of inflammatory myopathies: Comparison with clinical examination, magnetic resonance imaging and pathologic findings. *Br. J. Radiol.* **2016**, *89*, 20160283. [CrossRef] [PubMed]
13. Goo, M.; Johnston, L.M.; Hug, F.; Tucker, K. Systematic review of instrumented measures of skeletal muscle mechanical properties: Evidence for the application of Shear Wave Elastography with children. *Ultrasound Med. Biol.* **2020**, *46*, 1831–1840. [CrossRef] [PubMed]

14. Brandenburg, J.E.; Eby, S.F.; Song, P.; Zhao, H.; Landry, B.W.; Kingsley-Berg, S.; Bamlet, W.R.; Chen, S.; Sieck, G.C.; An, K.N. Feasibility and reliability of quantifying passive muscle stiffness in young children by using shear wave ultrasound elastography. *J. Ultrasound Med.* **2015**, *34*, 663–670. [CrossRef]
15. Liu, X.; Yu, H.K.; Sheng, S.Y.; Liang, S.M.; Lu, H.; Chen, R.Y.; Pan, M.; Wen, Z.B. Quantitative evaluation of passive muscle stiffness by shear wave elastography in healthy individuals of different ages. *Eur. Radiol.* **2020**, *31*, 3187–3194. [CrossRef]
16. Koppenhaver, S.L.; Scutella, D.; Sorrell, B.A.; Yahalom, J.; Fernández-de-las-Peñas, C.; Childs, J.D.; Shaffer, S.W.; Shinohara, M. Normative parameters and anthropometric variability of lumbar muscle stiffness using ultrasound shear-wave elastography. *Clin. Biomech.* **2019**, *62*, 113–120. [CrossRef] [PubMed]
17. Eby, S.F.; Cloud, B.A.; Brandenburg, J.E.; Giambini, H.; Song, P.; Chen, S.; LeBrasseur, N.K.; An, K.N. Shear wave elastography of passive skeletal muscle stiffness: Influences of sex and age throughout adulthood. *Clin. Biomech.* **2015**, *30*, 22–27. [CrossRef]
18. Zhang, L.; Yong, Q.; Pu, T.; Zheng, C.; Wang, M.; Shi, S.; Li, L. Grayscale ultrasonic and shear wave elastographic characteristics of the Achilles' tendon in patients with familial hypercholesterolemia: A pilot study. *Eur. J. Radiol.* **2018**, *109*, 1–7. [CrossRef]
19. Berko, N.S.; FitzGerald, E.F.; Amaral, T.D.; Payares, M.; Levin, T.L. Ultrasound elastography in children: Establishing the normal range of muscle elasticity. *Pediatr. Radiol.* **2014**, *44*, 158–163. [CrossRef]
20. Wenz, H.; Dieckmann, A.; Lehmann, T.; Brandl, U.; Mentzel, H.J. Strain ultrasound elastography of muscles in healthy children and healthy adults. *RoFo* **2019**, *191*, 1091–1098. [CrossRef]
21. Lacourpaille, L.; Hug, F.; Guével, A.; Péréon, Y.; Magot, A.; Hogrel, J.Y.; Nordez, A. Non-invasive assessment of muscle stiffness in patients with duchenne muscular dystrophy. *Muscle Nerve* **2015**, *51*, 284–286. [CrossRef]
22. Öztürk, M.; Sayinbatur, B. Real-time ultrasound elastography of the Achilles tendon in patients with cerebral palsy: Is there a correlation between strain ratio and biomechanical indicators? *J. Med. Ultrason.* **2018**, *45*, 143–148. [CrossRef]
23. Gennisson, J.L.; Deffieux, T.; Mace, E.; Montaldo, G.; Fink, M.; Tanter, M. Viscoelastic and anisotropic mechanical properties of in vivo muscle tissue assessed by supersonic shear imaging. *Ultrasound Med. Biol.* **2010**, *36*, 789–801. [CrossRef]
24. Brandenburg, J.E.; Eby, S.F.; Song, P.; Kingsley- Berg, S.; Bamlet, W.; Sieck, G.C.; An, K.N. Quantifying passive muscle stiffness in children with and without cerebral palsy using ultrasound shear wave elastography. *Dev. Med. Child Neurol.* **2016**, *176*, 1288–1294. [CrossRef]
25. Caliskan, E.; Akkoc, O.; Bayramoglu, Z.; Gozubuyuk, O.B.; Kural, D.; Azamat, S.; Adaletli, I. Effects of static stretching duration on muscle stiffness and blood flow in the rectus femoris in adolescents. *Med. Ultrason.* **2019**, *21*, 136–143. [CrossRef] [PubMed]
26. Lee, S.S.M.; Gaebler-Spira, D.; Zhang, L.; Rymer, W.Z.; Steele, K.M. Use of shear wave ultrasound elastography to quantify muscle properties in cerebral palsy. *Clin. Biomech.* **2016**, *31*, 20–28. [CrossRef]
27. Dağ, N.; Cerit, M.N.; Şendur, H.N.; Zinnuroğlu, M.; Muşmal, B.N.; Cindil, E.; Oktar, S.O. The utility of shear wave elastography in the evaluation of muscle stiffness in patients with cerebral palsy after botulinum toxin A injection. *Med. Ultrason.* **2020**, *47*, 609–615. [CrossRef]
28. Mansouri, M.; Birgani, P.M.; Kharazi, M.R.; Lotfian, M.; Naeimipoor, M.; Mirbagheri, M.M. Estimation of gait parameter using sonoelastography in children with cerebral palsy. In Proceedings of the 2016 38th Annual International Conference of the IEEE Engineering in Medicine and Biology Society (EMBC), Orlando, FL, USA, 16–20 August 2016; pp. 1729–1732. [CrossRef]
29. Linek, P.; Wolny, T.; Sikora, D.; Klepek, A. Supersonic shear imaging for quantification of lateral abdominal muscle shear modulus in pediatric population with scoliosis: A reliability and agreement study. *Ultrasound Med. Biol.* **2019**, *45*, 1551–1561. [CrossRef]
30. Saito, A.; Minagawa, H.; Watanabe, H.; Kawasaki, T.; Okada, K. Elasticity of the pronator teres muscle in youth baseball players with elbow injuries: Evaluation using ultrasound strain elastography. *J. Shoulder Elb. Surg.* **2018**, *27*, 1642–1649. [CrossRef] [PubMed]
31. Lee, S.Y.; Park, H.J.; Choi, Y.J.; Choi, S.H.; Kook, S.H.; Rho, M.H.; Chung, E.C. Value of adding sonoelastography to conven-tional ultrasound in patients with congenital muscular torticollis. *Pediatr. Radiol.* **2013**, *43*, 1566–1572. [CrossRef] [PubMed]
32. Lacourpaille, L.; Gross, R.; Hug, F.; Guével, A.; Péréon, Y.; Magot, A.; Hogrel, J.Y.; Nordez, A. Effects of Duchenne muscular dystrophy on muscle stiffness and response to electrically-induced muscle contraction: A 12-month follow-up. *Neuromuscul. Disord.* **2017**, *27*, 214–220. [CrossRef] [PubMed]
33. Kwon, D.R.; Park, G.Y.; Lee, S.U.; Chung, I. Spastic cerebral palsy in children: Dynamic sonoelastographic findings of medial gastrocnemius. *Radiology* **2012**, *263*, 794–801. [CrossRef]
34. Vola, E.A.; Albano, M.; Di Luise, C.; Servodidio, V.; Sansone, M.; Russo, S.; Corrado, B.; Servodio Iammarrone, C.; Caprio, M.G.; Vallone, G. Use of ultrasound shear wave to measure muscle stiffness in children with cerebral palsy. *J. Ultrasound* **2018**, *21*, 241–247. [CrossRef] [PubMed]
35. Bilgici, M.C.; Bekci, T.; Ulus, Y.; Ozyurek, H.; Aydin, O.F.; Tomak, L.; Selcuk, M.B. Quantitative assessment of muscular stiffness in children with cerebral palsy using acoustic radiation force impulse (ARFI) ultrasound elastography. *J. Med. Ultrason.* **2018**, *45*, 295–300. [CrossRef]
36. Lallemant-Dudek, P.; Vergari, C.; Dubois, G.; Forin, V.; Vialle, R.; Skalli, W. Ultrasound shearwave elas-tography to characterize muscles of healthy and cerebral palsy children. *Sci. Rep.* **2021**, *11*, 3577. [CrossRef]
37. Doruk Analan, P.; Aslan, H. Association between the elasticity of hip muscles and the hip migration index in cerebral palsy. *J. Ultrasound Med.* **2019**, *38*, 2667–2672. [CrossRef]
38. Park, G.Y.; Kwon, D.R. Sonoelastographic evaluation of medial gastrocnemius muscles intrinsic stiffness after rehabilitation therapy with botulinum toxin a injection in spastic cerebral palsy. *Arch. Phys. Med. Rehabil.* **2012**, *93*, 2085–2089. [CrossRef]

39. Bilgici, M.C.; Bekci, T.; Ulus, Y.; Bilgici, A.; Tomak, L.; Selcuk, M.B. Quantitative assessment of muscle stiffness with acoustic radiation force impulse elastography after botulinum toxin A injection in children with cerebral palsy. *J. Med. Ultrason.* **2018**, *45*, 137–141. [CrossRef] [PubMed]
40. Brandenburg, J.E.; Eby, S.F.; Song, P.; Bamlet, W.R.; Sieck, G.C.; An, K.N. Quantifying effect of onabotulinum toxin a on passive muscle stiffness in children with cerebral palsy using ultrasound shear wave elastography. *Am. J. Phys. Med. Rehabil.* **2018**, *97*, 500–506. [CrossRef]
41. Guo, R.; Xiang, X.; Qiu, L. Shear-wave elastography assessment of gluteal muscle contracture: Three case reports. *Medicine* **2018**, *97*, e13071. [CrossRef]
42. Li, A.; Peng, X.; Ma, Q.; Dong, Y.; Mao, C.; Hu, Y. Diagnostic performance of conventional ultrasound and quantitative and qualitative real-time shear wave elastography in musculoskeletal soft tissue tumors. *J. Orthop. Surg. Res.* **2020**, *15*, 103–107. [CrossRef] [PubMed]

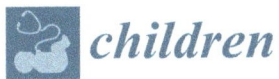 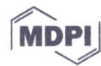

Article

Etiology of Carpal Tunnel Syndrome in a Large Cohort of Children

Christina T. Rüsch [1,2,†], Ursula Knirsch [1,†], Daniel M. Weber [3], Marianne Rohrbach [4], André Eichenberger [5], Jürg Lütschg [2], Kirsten Weber [6], Philip J. Broser [2] and Georg M. Stettner [1,*]

1. Neuromuscular Center Zurich and Department of Pediatric Neurology, University Children's Hospital Zurich, University of Zurich, 8032 Zurich, Switzerland; Christina.Ruesch@kispi.uzh.ch (C.T.R.); Ursula.Knirsch@kispi.uzh.ch (U.K.)
2. Division of Pediatric Neurology, Children's Hospital of Eastern Switzerland, 9006 St. Gallen, Switzerland; juerg.luetschg@unibas.ch (J.L.); PhilipJulian.Broser@kispisg.ch (P.J.B.)
3. Division of Hand Surgery, University Children's Hospital Zurich, University of Zurich, 8032 Zurich, Switzerland; Daniel.Weber@kispi.uzh.ch
4. Division of Metabolism, University Children's Hospital Zurich, University of Zurich, 8032 Zurich, Switzerland; Marianne.Rohrbach@kispi.uzh.ch
5. Division of Radiology, University Children's Hospital Zurich, University of Zurich, 8032 Zurich, Switzerland; Andre.Eichenberger@kispi.uzh.ch
6. Division of Hand Surgery, Children's Hospital of Eastern Switzerland, 9006 St. Gallen, Switzerland; kirsten.weber@kispisg.ch
* Correspondence: Georg.Stettner@kispi.uzh.ch; Tel.: +41-442-667-330
† These authors contributed equally to this work.

Abstract: (1) Background: Carpal tunnel syndrome (CTS), a compressive mononeuropathy of the median nerve at the wrist, is rare in childhood and occurs most frequently due to secondary causes. (2) Methods: Medical history, electrodiagnostic findings, and imaging data of patients with CTS from two pediatric neuromuscular centers were analyzed retrospectively. The etiology of CTS was investigated and compared with the literature. (3) Results: We report on a cohort of 38 CTS patients ($n = 22$ females, $n = 29$ bilateral, mean age at diagnosis 9.8 years). Electrodiagnostic studies of all patients revealed slowing of the antidromic sensory or orthodromic mixed nerve conduction velocities across the carpal tunnel or lack of the sensory nerve action potential and/or prolonged distal motor latencies. Median nerve ultrasound was diagnostic for CTS and confirmed tumorous and vascular malformations. Etiology was secondary in most patients ($n = 29$; 76%), and mucopolysaccharidosis was the most frequent underlying condition ($n = 14$; 37%). Idiopathic CTS was rare in this pediatric cohort ($n = 9$; 24%). (4) Conclusion: Since CTS in childhood is predominantly caused by an underlying disorder, a thorough evaluation and search for a causative condition is recommended in this age group.

Keywords: carpal tunnel syndrome; median nerve neuropathy; electrodiagnostic studies; neuromuscular ultrasound; mucopolysaccharidosis

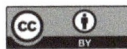

1. Introduction

Carpal tunnel syndrome (CTS) is a compressive mononeuropathy of the median nerve at the wrist. In contrast to CTS in adult patients, the condition in childhood is rare, often manifests with atypical symptoms, and most frequently occurs secondarily due to other causes. In children, CTS was first described by Martin and Mass in 1958 [1], who reported on three children with recurrent episodes of hand pain. In 1989 Poilvach [2] carried out an extensive literature search and presented 52 cases of childhood CTS. He suggested the first etiopathological classification of the various underlying causes. Van Meir and De Smet [3,4] continued this work and performed a meta-analysis of 163 cases from 35 articles, mostly case reports or small case series.

The diagnosis of CTS in adults is primarily based on clinical symptoms and can be confirmed with electrodiagnostic studies [5]. In children, symptoms are often atypical, which reinforces the importance of technical investigations. Regardless of the etiology, isolated slowing of sensory or mixed nerve conduction velocity and/or prolongation of the distal motor latency (DML) of the median nerve across the carpal tunnel are electrophysiological hallmarks for CTS. Recently, neuromuscular ultrasound has been recognized as a valuable method for different neuromuscular conditions including entrapment neuropathies. This applies also to the evaluation of CTS [6]. Characteristics of median nerve ultrasound studies consist of an increase of both the cross-sectional area (CSA) at the wrist and the wrist-to-forearm ratio (WFR) [6]. For the majority of pediatric CTS cases, an underlying cause can be found, in particular hereditary metabolic conditions with mucopolysaccharidoses and mucolipidoses as the largest disease group, followed by congenital malformations, connectivopathies, endocrinopathies, and acquired lesions like malignancies or tumor-like and traumatic lesions [2,3,7–9].

The aim of this study was to investigate the etiology of CTS in a cohort from two tertiary pediatric neuromuscular centers in Switzerland (University Children's Hospital Zurich and Children's Hospital of Eastern Switzerland St. Gallen, Switzerland). We retrospectively analyzed the data of pediatric patients with CTS and evaluated diagnostic procedures and findings.

2. Materials and Methods

We retrospectively analyzed data of patients diagnosed with CTS in two tertiary pediatric neuromuscular centers in Switzerland (University Children's Hospital Zurich and Children's Hospital of Eastern Switzerland St. Gallen). Patients with an age below 18 years at diagnosis of CTS with characteristic electrophysiological findings were included in our study. The main focus of this study was to investigate the etiology of childhood CTS. Therefore, demographic data, medical history, manifesting symptoms, examination findings, underlying conditions, and proportion of etiologies were analyzed. For identification of CTS patients, the clinical information system of the two participating centers and registers of electrophysiological and surgical interventions were screened for the diagnosis of CTS. All patients who were diagnosed with CTS in the years 2005–2020 at the University Children's Hospital Zurich and 2016–2020 at the Children's Hospital of Eastern Switzerland, St. Gallen were included. All patients gave their consent to be included in our study.

For inclusion, all patients had to fulfill standard electrodiagnostic criteria for CTS. Since this is a retrospective work, different electrophysiological standard procedures established for the investigation of adults were performed [10]. Midpalm stimulation of the median and ulnar nerves and determination of latency differences between the orthodromic mixed nerve potentials at the wrist at a distance of 6–8 cm was preferred, because this method is least dependent on the small size of the hand in younger children, in which standard distal distances used in other electrodiagnostic approaches sometimes cannot be respected. Any latency difference, referred to as "palmdiff", of ≥ 0.4 ms was considered diagnostic [10]. Alternatively, fractioned antidromic sensory nerve conduction studies with stimulation at the wrist and midpalm and recording of sensory nerve action potentials on the second digit were performed. Slowing of the sensory nerve conduction velocity of ≥ 10 m/s across the carpal tunnel was considered diagnostic for CTS. In addition, distal motor latencies (DML) of the compound muscle action potential (CMAP) recorded from the abductor pollicis brevis muscle were obtained after median nerve stimulation at the wrist with a distance of 7.0 cm whenever possible. A DML of ≥ 4.1 ms was considered diagnostic [10]. Two different ENMG systems were used in our centers: Viking Monograph (Nicolet Biomedical Inc. Madison, WI, USA; used in Zurich) and System Plus (Micromed, Venice, Italy; used in St. Gallen).

In addition, ultrasound imaging data of the median nerve were analyzed if available.

Median nerve ultrasound (US) imaging was done in 24% of the patients by a pediatric radiologist and/or pediatric neurologist trained in peripheral nerve US following standard procedures [6]. The presence of structural changes was investigated along the median nerve. In addition, the median nerve cross-sectional area (CSA) at standard locations was measured and the wrist-to-forearm ratio (WFR) calculated with reference to age related nerve US normal values [11,12]. In both centers a Canon Aplio i800 (Canon Medical Systems, Tokyo, Japan) ultrasound imaging system, equipped with i33LX9, i24LX8, i18LX5, and i22LH8 was used.

The study was approved by the local ethics committee on 23 June 2020, and registered with the Swiss project database (BASEC 2020-01016). Written informed consent was obtained from the caregivers prior to inclusion of participants in the study.

3. Results

3.1. Demographics

We identified 38 patients (n = 22 females, n = 16 males) diagnosed with CTS in the two pediatric neuromuscular centers between 2005 and 2020 in Zurich and 2016 and 2020 in St. Gallen. The demographics of the patients are shown in Table 1. See Supplementary Table S1 for more detailed individual information.

Table 1. Demographics of childhood CTS patients.

Gender [n (%)]	female	22 (58%)
	male	16 (42%)
Age at diagnosis [years]	mean	9.8
	range	2.5–17
Location [n (%)]	unilateral	9 (24%)
	bilateral	29 (76%)
Positive family history for CTS [n (%)]		8 (21%)
Treatment [n (%)]	conservative	11 (29%)
	surgical	27 (71%)

3.2. Etiology

Lysosomal storage diseases (mucopolysaccharidosis and mucolipidosis) were the most frequent underlying conditions in our cohort (n = 15; 39%). Five patients (13%) showed CTS associated with a hereditary neuropathy (n = 3 probable hereditary neuropathy with liability to pressure palsy (HNPP) with positive family history, n = 1 Charcot-Marie-Tooth CMT type 1A, n = 1 associated with autosomal recessive spastic ataxia of Charlevoix-Saguenay (ARSACS)). In the three patients with a positive family history for HNPP the parents did not consent to genetic testing for their children. We identified CTS due to congenital malformations in four patients (11%). Two of them had been diagnosed with geleophysic dysplasia, one with the ultra-rare condition melorheostosis and one with a hemihypertrophia syndrome of unknown etiology. In two patients (5%), CTS occurred due to a benign tumor (n = 2 perineurioma, Figure 1), of which one perineurioma was associated with a PIK3CA gene mutation. A posttraumatic CTS was found in two patients (5%). One patient (3%) suffered from bilateral CTS associated with rheumatoid arthritis. Altogether, a secondary CTS etiology was confirmed in 29 patients (76%). In only nine patients (24%) was CTS considered idiopathic because of the absence of other explaining findings. See Table 2 for a summary of the CTS etiology.

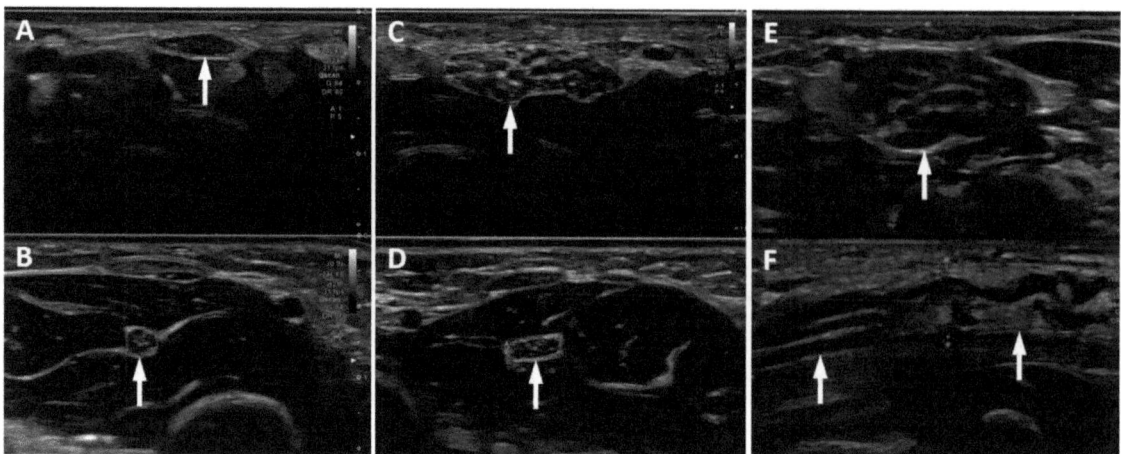

Figure 1. Ultrasound of the median nerve in childhood CTS. (**A,B**) Idiopathic CTS with transverse sonogram of the median nerve at wrist (**A**) and forearm (**B**). The median nerve ultrasound investigation demonstrated a pathologically increased WFR of 2.3. (**C–F**) Intraneural perineurioma in two patients: Transverse sonograms of the median nerve at wrist (**C**) and forearm (**D**) of one patient, and transverse (**E**) and longitudinal (**F**) sonogram at the wrist of the second patient with intraneural perineurioma.

Table 2. Etiology of CTS.

		Number of Patients (n)	Unilateral vs. Bilateral
Lysosomal storage diseases	MPS Type 1	4	bilateral
	MPS Type 2	7	bilateral
	MPS Type 3	1	bilateral
	MPS Type 6	2	bilateral
	Mucolipidosis Type 3	1	bilateral
Neuropathy	HNPP (assumed)	3	bilateral
	CMT1A	1	bilateral
	associated with ARSACS	1	bilateral
Congenital malformation	Geleophysic dysplasia	2	bilateral
	Melorheostosis	1	unilateral
	Hemihypertrophia	1	bilateral
Tumor	Intraneural Perineurioma	2	unilateral
Traumatic lesion		2	unilateral
Rheumatoid arthritis		1	bilateral
Idiopathic		9	4 unilateral, 5 bilateral

ARSACS = autosomal recessive spastic ataxia of Charlevoix-Saguenay; CMT1A = Charcot-Marie-Tooth disease type 1A; HNPP = hereditary neuropathy with liability to pressure palsy; MPS = mucopolysaccharidosis.

3.3. Clinical Findings

Most patients indicated typical complaints of a CTS, e.g., paraesthesia and/or dysaesthesia. However, only 29% (4/14) of CTS patients with MPS indicated complaints related to the CTS, although thenar muscle atrophy was already present at diagnosis in 86% (12/14) of these patients. Thenar muscle atrophy was also present at the time of diagnosis of CTS at a high proportion in most of the other conditions: congenital malformations 3/4, tumors 2/2, traumatic lesion 1/2, rheumatoid arthritis 1/1. Only in CTS associated with neuropathy was thenar muscle atrophy not observed (0/5), and idiopathic CTS showed thenar muscle atrophy only in 3/9 patients. See Supplementary Table S1 for more detailed individual information.

3.4. Electrophysiological Examination

Electrodiagnostic studies of all patients revealed a significant latency difference between orthodromic median and ulnar mixed nerve potentials and/or slowing of the antidromic median sensory nerve conduction velocities across the carpal tunnel or lack of the sensory nerve action potential and/or prolonged median DML. See Supplementary Table S1 for detailed information.

3.5. Ultrasound Imaging

In nine patients US imaging was performed. In all CTS patients, the WFR ratio and/or the CSA of the median nerve at the wrist was increased. In addition, structural lesions of the median nerve were reliably detected. See Supplementary Table S1 for details. In the two patients with perineurioma, the echogenicity and structure of the nerve was altered (enlarged fascicles, increased perineuronal tissue). In these patients an MRI of the wrist and forearm was also performed and confirmed the US findings. The final diagnosis was then confirmed by histological examination following incisional biopsy during surgical decompression of the carpal tunnel.

4. Discussion

Compared to CTS in adults, CTS in children is rare. However, since children may not present with typical symptoms and may, in part, not communicate their complaints depending on their developmental stage and/or cognitive impairment, CTS is possibly underdiagnosed in this age group. Nevertheless, it is important to consider the presence of CTS even in toddlers with atypical symptoms, because the majority of CTS is caused by an underlying condition and requires early surgical treatment in order to prevent axonal median nerve damage.

In our cohort the age range at diagnosis was 2.5 to 17 years. The youngest child reported with CTS was 9 months old [13]. CTS was bilateral in 76% of our cohort, and a bilateral manifestation occurred mostly in CTS with an underlying hereditary disorder. In comparison, bilateral CTS at manifestation occurs only in approximately 50% of the adult population [14]. A surgical intervention was performed in 71% of our cohort. This high rate of surgical interventions was also related to the secondary nature of childhood CTS. Almost all children from our cohort who harbored a hereditary condition (e.g., lysosomal storage diseases, congenital malformations) or a tumor associated with CTS required surgical intervention because of the low likelihood of improvement under conservative treatment due to the stationary or progressive nature of these conditions.

Mucopolysaccharidosis was the most common cause of CTS in our cohort. A high prevalence of mucopolysaccharidosis in childhood CTS is also reported in the literature [3,8,15]. MPS constitutes a group of rare lysosomal storage diseases with multisystem manifestation. CTS is a common musculoskeletal manifestation of MPS [9,16–18]. The symptoms of CTS in patients with MPS are, however, often not as distinct as in other etiologies. In our cohort, less than 30% indicated complaints related to CTS. The early nonspecific symptoms of CTS in MPS, compounded with communication barriers due to age and intellectual disability, often lead to delayed diagnosis with thenar wasting and potential permanent loss of hand function [17,18]. Therefore, routine biannual physical examination and annual electrophysiological screening for CTS is recommended in the care standards for MPS even in the absence of suggestive symptoms [17]. Adhering to this recommendation, CTS was diagnosed in MPS patients at an early stage in our cohort, and surgical intervention was performed in all MPS CTS patients. Three of 14 MPS patients showed recurrent CTS within 3–11 years after the first surgical intervention. Follow up investigations showed normalization of the nerve conduction studies only in three patients after carpal tunnel release. These three patients were identified and treated very early (below 5 years of age). The patients with a later surgical intervention showed chronic axonal damage of the median nerve. These findings confirm the importance of physical examinations every six months and annual electrodiagnostic screening, which enables early diagnosis and treatment of CTS in the MPS population. As reviewed by Patel et al. [17], MPS patients are at risk of developing CTS very early in life. In fact, the youngest patient from our cohort, diagnosed with CTS at 30 months of age, belongs to the MPS patient group. Screening for CTS, therefore, should be initiated immediately after the diagnosis of MPS and continued frequently thereafter.

Polyneuropathy was the reason for CTS in five patients (13%) in our cohort. One patient suffered from CMT1A and one patient from sensorimotor neuropathy associated with ARSACS. In one patient, HNPP was assumed as causative for CTS because of a genetically confirmed HNPP in the child's mother. Two additional patients with early onset CTS were siblings, and family history revealed the presence of HNPP over several generations. The parents of these three patients did not consent to the genetic confirmation of HNPP in their children. Del Colle [19] describes an identical constellation compared to the family with two affected siblings in our cohort: A family with HNPP in several generations and a high prevalence of early onset CTS, in some cases as the only manifestation of the HNPP. In general, bilaterally prolonged DML of the median nerve, prolonged DML and/or reduced motor nerve conduction velocities in the peroneal nerve and sensory nerve conduction velocity slowing are highly suggestive of HNPP when there is a positive family history of polyneuropathy [20].

CTS associated with congenital malformations was the fourth most common etiology in our cohort (affecting 11%). Our cohort includes one individual with melorheostosis, an extremely rare and progressive bone disease accompanied by hyperostosis and soft tissue fibrosis. Hand involvement had only been reported sporadically in this condition [21–23]. Interestingly, our cohort also includes two patients with geleophysic dysplasia, a rare hereditary condition characterized by severe short stature, short extremities, progressive joint limitation, thickened skin, and pseudomuscular build. Together with acromicric dysplasia, the geleophysic dysplasia belongs to the acromelic dysplasia group. These two conditions share, in part, similarities of the genetic pathway and phenotype. Hand involvement causes an increased risk for the development of CTS, which might be as high as 35% in geleophysic and acromicric dysplasias [24].

In our cohort we found two patients with an intraneural perineurioma, a rare benign peripheral nerve sheath tumor, which has only been included in the WHO classification system since 2000 [25]. In both patients the diagnosis of the tumor was suspected in the US investigation which followed the electrophysiological diagnosis of CTS. A histopathological examination confirmed the diagnosis in these two patients. Molecular investigation performed with biopsy material showed a pathogenic somatic mutation in the PIK3CA gene in one patient. Perineuriomatous pseudo-onion bulb proliferation is considered part of the PIK3CA-related overgrowth spectrum (PROS) [26] and has also been described in lipomatosis of peripheral nerves with or without nerve territory overgrowth in association with PIK3CA mutations [27]. Dailiana et al. [28] published a case series of tumors and tumor-like lesions affecting the median nerve as rare causes for CTS. However, most of the patients in this study showed nerve compression due to extraneural masses.

In nine patients (24%), the CTS was classified as idiopathic and no obvious underlying condition could be confirmed. This etiological group included one child with a bilateral CTS and the additional diagnosis of familial Mediterranean fever (FMF), who was under colchicine treatment for 18 months prior to the manifestation of bilateral CTS. Since it is known that colchicine can cause polyneuropathies amongst other side effects, Isikay et al. [29] examined a group of 88 children with FMF under Colchicine treatment and found only one patient with CTS. In addition, only Bademci et al. [30] described a bilateral CTS in a young woman with FMF. Due to the fact of the high incidence of both FMF in some populations and CTS in general, this association might be random, which is also the conclusion of a large retrospective study of comorbidities in 2000 FMF patients including more than 600 children [31]. Our patient with bilateral CTS and FMF might nevertheless be an example for the suspicion that even the low proportion of idiopathic CTS in children might be overestimated, because this etiological group most likely includes patients with underlying disorders that are unknown or not detectable at the time of CTS manifestation.

Neuromuscular US is becoming a standard investigation in the evaluation of peripheral nerve and muscle diseases, including CTS. In addition to electrodiagnostic procedures, detection of median nerve enlargement at the wrist by US has been suggested as a sensitive and valuable diagnostic method [32–34]. Billakota et al. [6] performed a large retrospective analysis of median nerve ultrasound investigations in CTS and concluded that median nerve US is nearly as sensitive as electrophysiological testing, which is considered the diagnostic gold standard in CTS. Bäumer et al. [35] specifically examined the value of US in the management of patients with MPS. In their study, US had an even higher sensitivity for the detection of CTS compared to electrophysiology. In our cohort, which focused on the etiology and not on the diagnostic measures, US was performed only in a small number of patients. This is primarily a consequence of the retrospective nature of this study. Even the low number of median nerve US investigations in our cohort, however, demonstrates that the increase of both the CSA of the median nerve at the wrist and the WFR are also indicative of CTS in children. In addition, nerve US is a sensitive method to detect tumor associated median nerve lesions. Therefore, US is a valuable tool to support the clinical and electrophysiological diagnosis of CTS, especially in children since it is a quick, non-invasive and painless method.

In conclusion, we were able to identify a broad spectrum of underlying etiologies in our cohort of childhood CTS. Our study confirms that idiopathic CTS in children is rare and most commonly secondary to an underlying condition with mucopolysaccharidosis as the most common cause.

To prevent delayed diagnosis, which can lead to thenar wasting and permanent loss of hand function, we propose the following diagnostic algorithm for patients at risk and patients with symptoms suggestive of CTS:

Patients with conditions associated with a high risk for CTS should be clinically screened for symptoms of CTS at the time of the primary diagnosis and frequently thereafter. Thenar muscle atrophy, pain and/or sensory symptoms, and/or disturbances of nail growth in digits I to III, a positive Tinel sign at the wrist and/or deterioration of dexterity are features potentially pointing to the presence of CTS. Physical examination is recommended as frequent as every 6 months for MPS patients, the largest patient group at risk for CTS [17,18]. In addition to lysosomal storage diseases, several genetic conditions, including HNPP and other hereditary neuropathies and congenital malformation syndromes like acromelic dysplasia, melorheostasis, and hemihypertrophia syndromes have a high risk for early CTS, too, and should also be screened for CTS by frequent physical examination. It is, however, important to emphasize, that CTS symptoms in children are often atypical and complaints might not be communicated due to the developmental stage and/or cognitive impairment of these patients. Therefore, physical examination and screening for CTS should be supplemented by median nerve US. Our study shows that the early conduct of median nerve US might be diagnostic for childhood CTS. In addition, all patients at risk should undergo annual or even more frequent electrodiagnostic investigations, applying standard procedures for the investigation of CTS. If these investigations prove the presence of CTS, early surgical intervention should be discussed because conservative treatment might not be effective due to the stationary or progressive nature of the primary conditions and the high risk of axonal median nerve damage.

Patients with symptoms suggestive of CTS without known underlying conditions should undergo the same procedures consisting of physical examination, median nerve US, and electrodiagnostic testing. Due to the frequent secondary nature of childhood CTS, a thorough investigation and search for an underlying disease is mandatory.

Supplementary Materials: The following are available online at https://www.mdpi.com/article/10.3390/children8080624/s1, Table S1: Demographics, etiology, and clinical and diagnostic findings of childhood CTS.

Author Contributions: Conceptualization, C.T.R., U.K., P.J.B. and G.M.S.; data collection and analysis, C.T.R., U.K., M.R. and G.M.S.; clinical investigations, all authors; electrodiagnostic investigations, U.K., J.L., P.J.B. and G.M.S.; US investigations, A.E. and P.J.B.; surgical treatment D.M.W. and K.W.; writing—original draft preparation, C.T.R., U.K. and G.M.S.; writing—review and editing, all authors; funding acquisition, G.M.S. All authors have read and agreed to the published version of the manuscript.

Funding: This study was supported by a training fellowship granted by the Swiss Muscle Society to CT Rüsch.

Institutional Review Board Statement: The study was approved by the local ethics committee on 23 June 2020, and registered with the Swiss project database (BASEC 2020-01016).

Informed Consent Statement: Written informed consent was obtained from the caregivers of all subjects prior to inclusion of participants in the study.

Data Availability Statement: Data is contained within the article or Supplementary Material.

Acknowledgments: We thank all patients and caregivers for their participation in this study.

Conflicts of Interest: The authors declare no conflict of interest. The sponsor had no role in the design, execution, interpretation, or writing of the study.

References

1. Martin, C.; Masse, P. Carpal tunnel syndrome in children. *Arch. Fr. Pediatr.* **1958**, *15*, 930–940. [PubMed]
2. Poilvache, P.; Carlier, A.; Rombouts, J.J.; Partoune, E.; Lejeune, G. Carpal tunnel syndrome in childhood: Report of five new cases. *J. Pediatr. Orthop.* **1989**, *9*, 687–690. [CrossRef]
3. Van Meir, N.; Smet, L. Carpal tunnel syndrome in children. *Acta Orthop. Belg.* **2003**, *69*, 387–395. [CrossRef]
4. Van Meir, N.; Smet, L. Carpal tunnel syndrome in children. *J. Pediatr. Orthop. B* **2005**, *14*, 42–45. [CrossRef]
5. Deymeer, F.; Jones, H.R., Jr. Pediatric median mononeuropathies: A clinical and electromyographic study. *Muscle Nerve* **1994**, *17*, 755–762. [CrossRef]
6. Billakota, S.; Hobson-Webb, L.D. Standard median nerve ultrasound in carpal tunnel syndrome: A retrospective review of 1021 cases. *Clin. Neurophysiol. Pract.* **2017**, *2*, 188–191. [CrossRef]
7. Dabaj, I.; Gitiaux, C.; Avila-Smirnow, D.; Ropers, J.; Desguerre, I.; Salon, A.; Pannier, S.; Tebani, A.; Valayannopoulos, V.; Quijano-Roy, S. Diagnosis and management of carpal tunnel syndrome in children with mucopolysaccharidosis: A 10 year experience. *Diagnostics* **2020**, *10*, 5. [CrossRef] [PubMed]
8. Leti Acciaro, A.; Pilla, F.; Faldini, C.; Adani, R. The carpal tunnel syndrome in children. *Musculoskelet. Surg.* **2018**, *102*, 261–265. [CrossRef]
9. Viskochil, D.; Muenzer, J.; Guffon, N.; Garin, C.; Munoz-Rojas, M.V.; Moy, K.A.; Hutchinson, D.T. Carpal tunnel syndrome in mucopolysaccharidosis I: A registry-based cohort study. *Dev. Med. Child Neurol.* **2017**, *59*, 1269–1275. [CrossRef]
10. Werner, R.A.; Andary, M. Electrodiagnostic evaluation of carpal tunnel syndrome. *Muscle Nerve* **2011**, *44*, 597–607. [CrossRef]
11. Druzhinin, D.; Naumova, E.; Nikitin, S. Nerve ultrasound normal values in children and young adults. *Muscle Nerve* **2019**, *60*, 757–761. [CrossRef] [PubMed]
12. Jenny, C.; Lütschg, J.; Broser, P.J. Change in cross-sectional area of the median nerve with age in neonates, infants and children analyzed by high-resolution ultrasound imaging. *Eur. J. Paediatr. Neurol.* **2020**, *29*, 137–143. [CrossRef] [PubMed]
13. Algahtani, H.; Watson, B.V.; Thomson, J.; Al-Rabia, M.W. Idiopathic bilateral carpal tunnel syndrome in a 9-month-old infant presenting as a pseudo-dystonia. *Pediatr. Neurol.* **2014**, *51*, 147–150. [CrossRef] [PubMed]
14. Bland, J.D.P.; Rudolfer, S.M. Clinical surveillance of carpal tunnel syndrome in two areas of the United Kingdom, 1991–2001. *J. Neurol. Neurosurg. Psychiatry* **2003**, *74*, 1674–1679. [CrossRef]
15. Lamberti, P.M.; Light, T.R. Carpal tunnel syndrome in children. *Hand Clin.* **2002**, *18*, 331–337. [CrossRef]
16. Kwon, J.Y.; Ko, K.; Sohn, Y.B.; Kim, S.J.; Park, S.W.; Kim, S.H.; Cho, S.Y.; Jin, D.K. High prevalence of carpal tunnel syndrome in children with mucopolysaccharidosis type II (Hunter syndrome). *Am. J. Med. Genet. Part A* **2011**, *155*, 1329–1335. [CrossRef]
17. Patel, P.; Antoniou, G.; Clark, D.; Ketteridge, D.; Williams, N. Screening for Carpal Tunnel Syndrome in Patients with Mucopolysaccharidosis. *J. Child Neurol.* **2020**, *35*, 410–417. [CrossRef]
18. White, K.; Kim, T.; Neufeld, J.A. Clinical assessment and treatment of carpal tunnel syndrome in the mucopolysaccharidoses. *J. Pediatr. Rehabil. Med.* **2010**, *3*, 57–62. [CrossRef]

19. Del Colle, R.; Fabrizi, G.M.; Turazzini, M.; Cavallaro, T.; Silvestri, M.; Rizzuto, N. Hereditary neuropathy with liability to pressure palsies: Electrophysiological and genetic study of a family with carpal tunnel syndrome as only clinical manifestation. *Neurol. Sci.* **2003**, *24*, 57–60. [CrossRef]
20. Leguern, E.; Gugenheim, M.; Maisonobe, T.; Léger, J.M.; Vallat, J.M.; Agid, Y.; Bouche, P.; Brice, A. Clinical, electrophysiologic, and molecular correlations in 13 families with hereditary neuropathy with liability to pressure palsies and a chromosome 17~11.2 deletion. *Neurology* **1995**, *45*, 2018–2023.
21. Abdullah, S.; Nor, N.F.M.; Haflah, N.H.M. Melorheostosis of the hand affecting the c6 sclerotome and presenting with carpal tunnel syndrome. *Singap. Med. J.* **2014**, *55*, 54–56. [CrossRef] [PubMed]
22. Ameen, S.; Nagy, L.; Gerich, U.; Anderson, S.E. Melorheostosis of the hand with complicating bony spur formation and bursal inflammation: Diagnosis and treatment. *Skelet. Radiol.* **2002**, *31*, 467–470. [CrossRef]
23. Suresh, S.; Muthukumar, T.; Saifuddin, A. Classical and unusual imaging appearances of melorheostosis. *Clin. Radiol.* **2010**, *65*, 593–600. [CrossRef]
24. Marzin, P.; Thierry, B.; Dancasius, A.; Cavau, A.; Michot, C.; Rondeau, S.; Baujat, G.; Phan, G.; Bonnière, M.; Le Bourgeois, M.; et al. Geleophysic and acromicric dysplasias: Natural history, genotype–phenotype correlations, and management guidelines from 38 cases. *Genet. Med.* **2021**, *23*, 331–340. [CrossRef]
25. Scheller, C.; Richter, H.P.; Scheuerle, A.; Kretschmer, T.; König, R.W.; Antoniadis, G. Intraneural perineuriomas; a rare entity. Clinical, surgical and neuropathological details in the management of these lesions. *Zentralbl. Neurochir.* **2008**, *69*, 134–138. [CrossRef]
26. Koutlas, I.G.; Anbinder, A.-L.; Alshagroud, R.; Rodrigues Cavalcante, A.S.; Al Kindi, M.; Crenshaw, M.M.; Sapp, J.C.; Kondolf, H.; Lindhurst, M.J.; Dudley, J.N.; et al. Orofacial overgrowth with peripheral nerve enlargement and perineuriomatous pseudo-onion bulb proliferations is part of the PIK3CA-related overgrowth spectrum. *Hum. Genet. Genom. Adv.* **2020**, *1*, 100009. [CrossRef]
27. Blackburn, P.R.; Milosevic, D.; Marek, T.; Folpe, A.L.; Howe, B.M.; Spinner, R.J.; Carter, J.M. PIK3CA mutations in lipomatosis of nerve with or without nerve territory overgrowth. *Mod. Pathol.* **2020**, *33*, 420–430. [CrossRef] [PubMed]
28. Dailiana, Z.H.; Bougioukli, S.; Varitimidis, S.; Kontogeorgakos, V.; Togia, E.; Vlychou, M.; Malizos, K.N. Tumors and tumor-like lesions mimicking carpal tunnel syndrome. *Arch. Orthop. Trauma Surg.* **2014**, *134*, 139–144. [CrossRef] [PubMed]
29. Işıkay, S.; Yılmaz, K.; Yiğiter, R.; Balat, A.; Büyükçelik, M. Colchicine treatment in children with familial Mediterranean fever: Is it a risk factor for neuromyopathy? *Pediatr. Neurol.* **2013**, *49*, 417–419. [CrossRef]
30. Bademci, G.; Erdemoglu, A.K.; Evliyaoglu, C.; Atasoy, P.; Keskil, S. Bilateral carpal tunnel syndrome associated to familial Mediterranean fever. *Clin. Neurol. Neurosurg.* **2005**, *108*, 77–79. [CrossRef]
31. Balcı-Peynircioğlu, B.; Kaya-Akça, Ü.; Arıcı, Z.S.; Avcı, E.; Yeliz Akkaya-Ulum, Z.; Karadağ, Ö.; Kalyoncu, U.; Bilginer, Y.; Yılmaz, E.; Özen, S. Comorbidities in familial Mediterranean fever: Analysis of 2000 genetically confirmed patients. *Rheumatology* **2020**, *59*, 1372–1380. [CrossRef] [PubMed]
32. Beekman, R.; Visser, L.H. Sonography in the diagnosis of carpal tunnel syndrome: A critical review of the literature. *Muscle Nerve* **2003**, *27*, 26–33. [CrossRef] [PubMed]
33. Duncan, I.; Sullivan, P.; Lomas, F. Sonography in the diagnosis of carpal tunnel syndrome. *AJR Am. J. Roentgenol.* **1999**, *3*, 681–684. [CrossRef]
34. Mhoon, J.T.; Juel, V.C.; Hobson-Webb, L.D. Median nerve ultrasound as a screening tool in carpal tunnel syndrome: Correlation of cross-sectional area measures with electrodiagnostic abnormality. *Muscle Nerve* **2012**, *46*, 871–878. [CrossRef] [PubMed]
35. Bäumer, T.; Bühring, N.; Schelle, T.; Münchau, A.; Muschol, N. Nerve ultrasound in clinical management of carpal tunnel syndrome in mucopolysaccharidosis. *Dev. Med. Child Neurol.* **2016**, *58*, 1172–1179. [CrossRef]

Article

Two Approaches for a Genetic Analysis of Pompe Disease: A Literature Review of Patients with Pompe Disease and Analysis Based on Genomic Data from the General Population

Kyung-Sun Park

Department of Laboratory Medicine, Kyung Hee University School of Medicine and Kyung Hee University Medical Center, Seoul 02447, Korea; drkyungsun@gmail.com or drparkkyungsun@khu.ac.kr; Tel.: +82-2-958-8674

Abstract: In this study, two different approaches were applied in the analysis of the *GAA* gene. One was analyzed based on patients with Pompe disease, and the other was analyzed based on *GAA* genomic data from unaffected carriers in a general population genetic database. For this, *GAA* variants in Korean and Japanese patients reported in previous studies and in patients reported in the Pompe disease *GAA* variant database were analyzed as a model. In addition, *GAA* variants in the Korean Reference Genome Database (KRGDB), the Japanese Multi Omics Reference Panel (jMorp), and the Genome Aggregation Database (gnomAD) were analyzed. Overall, approximately 50% of the pathogenic or likely pathogenic variants (PLPVs) found in unaffected carriers were also found in real patients with Pompe disease (Koreans, 57.1%; Japanese, 46.2%). In addition, there was a moderate positive correlation (Spearman's correlation coefficient of 0.45–0.69) between the proportion of certain PLPVs in patients and the minor allele frequency of their variants in a general population database. Based on the analysis of general population databases, the total carrier frequency for Pompe disease in Koreans and Japanese was estimated to be 1.7% and 0.7%, respectively, and the predicted genetic prevalence was 1:13,657 and 1:78,013, respectively.

Keywords: Pompe disease; *GAA* gene; general population database; carrier frequency; genetic prevalence

1. Introduction

Pompe disease, or glycogen storage disease type II (MIM #232300), is a monogenic autosomal recessive disorder caused by deficiency of lysosomal alpha-glucosidase (GAA). This deficiency results in the accumulation of lysosomal glycogen in various body tissues, especially in cardiac and skeletal muscles [1–3]. Pompe patients who develop hypertrophic cardiomyopathy and general muscle weakness within the first year of life are classified as having classic infantile Pompe disease. Without enzyme replacement therapy (ERT), classic infantile Pompe disease is typically fatal within the first year of life. Nonclassic Pompe disease (or late-onset Pompe disease (LOPD) or childhood or adult onset Pompe disease) [3] is associated with a slowly progressive weakness of proximal muscles and respiratory dysfunction. Patients with nonclassic Pompe disease either develop symptoms without cardiac involvement before 1 year of life or develop symptoms after the first year of life. Given the benefits of early diagnosis and treatment with ERT, Pompe disease was included in the recommended uniform screening panel (the newborn screening program, NBS) in the USA [4].

In general, a research on rare diseases is conducted with the clinical and genetic information of patients. However, a huge amount of genetic information has been released to public databases, allowing us to think of new approaches to genetic diseases. Theoretically, the prevalence of a specific Mendelian disease is estimated by analyzing the proportion of unaffected carriers (carrier frequency) with the genomic information in the general population. In this study, two approaches were applied in the analysis of Pompe disease. One was based on the literature review of patients with Pompe disease reported, and the other was based on the genomic information from the general population. For these, the *GAA* gene in patients and the general population was analyzed.

2. Materials and Methods

2.1. Analysis Workflow

The entire analysis workflow for the two approaches is presented in Figure 1. A literature search for Korean and Japanese patients with Pompe disease was conducted, and the causative *GAA* variants in the patients were analyzed. In this study, newborn cases without specific symptoms or signs were excluded from the analysis. For the *GAA* analysis in unaffected carriers, the *GAA* gene from both Korean and Japanese general population databases was analyzed. Recently, a database containing Korean genomic information was released, called the Korean Reference Genome Database (KRGDB, http://coda.nih.go.kr/coda/KRGDB/index.jsp, accessed on 8 February 2021), which contains 1722 Korean genomic data [5]. In the present study, *GAA* genetic variants found in KRGDB (30× coverage group, 1465 individuals) were analyzed. In addition, the Japanese Multi Omics Reference Panel (jMorp, https://jmorp.megabank.tohoku.ac.jp/202102/variants, accessed on 16 March 2021) was used to analyze *GAA* variants in the Japanese general population [6,7]. To date, the jMorp database contains the genomic data (whole-genome sequencing data) of 8380 Japanese individuals.

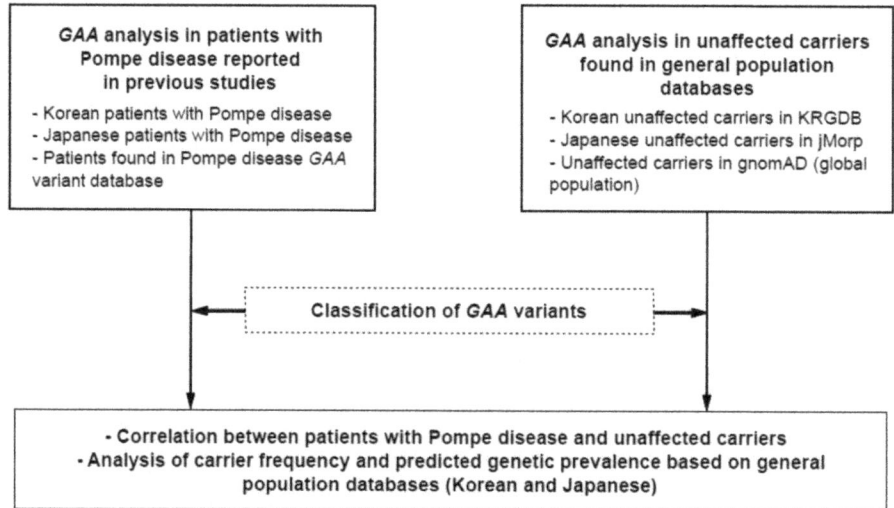

Figure 1. Analysis workflow in this study. The Pompe disease *GAA* variant database (http://www.pompevariantdatabase.nl/) was accessed on 16 March 2021, KRGDB (http://coda.nih.go.kr/coda/KRGDB/index.jsp) was accessed on 8 February 2021, jMorp (https://jmorp.megabank.tohoku.ac.jp/202102/variants) was accessed on 16 March 2021, and gnomAD (https://gnomad.broadinstitute.org/) was accessed on 17 March 2021.

In order to compare *GAA* variants between general databases, excluding common variants, *GAA* variants with a minor allele frequency (MAF) < 1% in East Asians in the Genome Aggregation Database (gnomAD, https://gnomad.broadinstitute.org/, accessed on 17 March 2021, search by genomic region: chr17:78,075,380-78,093,680 (GRCh37/hg19)) [8] were compared with those in KRGDB and JMorp. For a comparison between patients with Pompe disease and the general population, *GAA* variants in Korean or Japanese patients were compared with those found in KRGDB or JMorp. In addition, *GAA* variants in the Pompe disease *GAA* variant database [9] (http://www.pompevariantdatabase.nl/, accessed on 16 March 2021) were compared with those in the general population (global) in gnomAD (https://gnomad.broadinstitute.org/, accessed on 17 March 2021). A Venn diagram for comparative analysis used InteractiVenn [10] (Figure 2). A correlation between the proportions of certain PLPVs among all PLPVs found in total patients considering the frequency of detection (for simplicity, the proportions of certain PLPVs) and the MAF of those variants in a general population database was analyzed using Spearman's rank correlation analysis. To determine the clinical severity of Pompe disease per specific *GAA* variant, information provided by the Pompe disease *GAA* variant database was used [9] (http://www.pompevariantdatabase.nl/, accessed on 16 March 2021).

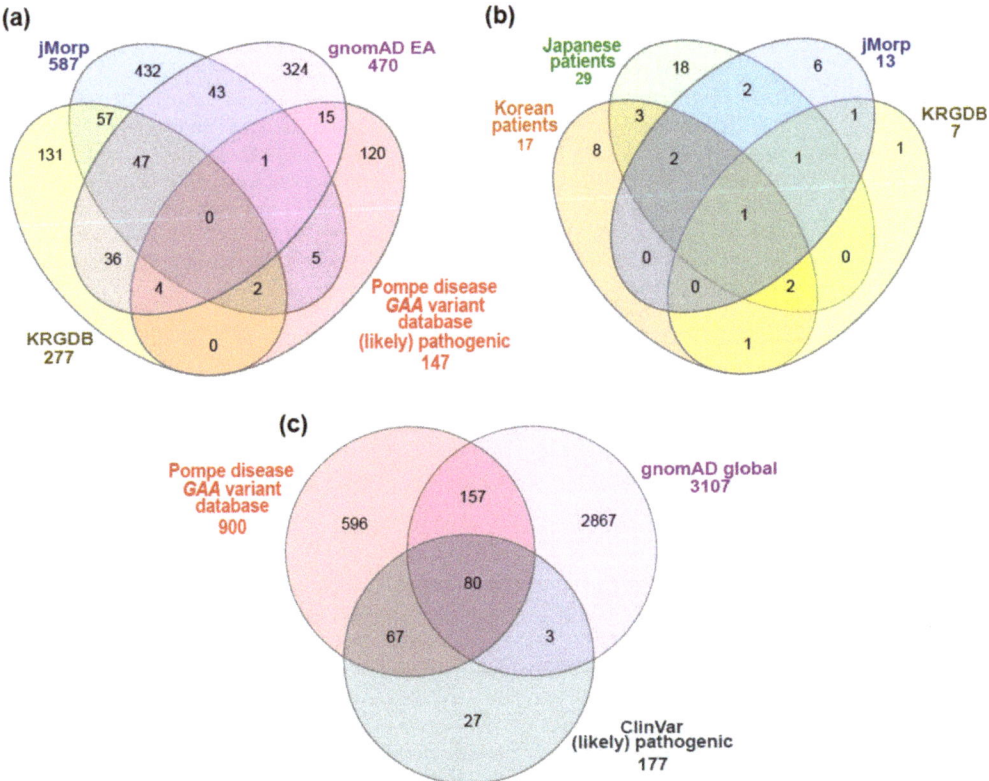

Figure 2. *GAA* variants found in patients with Pompe disease or in general population databases. (**a**) Number of *GAA* variants with MAF < 1% in general population databases (KRGDB, jMorp, and gnomAD) (East Asian) and number of (likely) pathogenic variants (with a review status of ≥2 gold stars in ClinVar) in the Pompe disease *GAA* variant database; (**b**) comparison of (likely) pathogenic variants found in Korean or Japanese patients, KRGDB, and jMorp; and (**c**) number of *GAA* variants in the Pompe disease *GAA* variant database, number of *GAA* variant with MAF < 1% in gnomAD (global), and number of (likely) pathogenic variants with a review status of ≥2 gold stars in ClinVar.

2.2. GAA Variant Classification

All *GAA* variants were analyzed based on NM_000152.5 (NP_000143.2) and described following the Human Genome Variation Society (HGVS) variant nomenclature standards ((http://varnomen.hgvs.org/, accessed on 17 March 2021). The *GAA* variants described in an incorrect nomenclature, which were reported in the previous literature, were not included in this study. The *GAA* variants in KRGDB, jMorp, and previous literature on Korean or Japanese patients with Pompe disease were classified or reclassified according to the 2015 American College of Medical Genetics and Genomics and the Association for Molecular Pathology standards and guidelines (2015 ACMG/AMP guidelines) [11] and specifications by a ClinGen lysosomal storage disorders expert panel (https://clinicalgenome.org/affiliation/50009/, accessed on 20 March 2021). Briefly, the PVS1, PS1, PS3, PM2, PM5, and PP4 ACMG/AMP variant criteria by the ClinGen lysosomal storage disorders expert panel (https://clinicalgenome.org/affiliation/50009/, accessed on 20 March 2021) were applied. The PM3 criterion was applied following a general recommendation by the Sequence Variant Interpretation Working Group (https://clinicalgenome.org/working-groups/sequence-variant-interpretation/, accessed on 20 March 2021); that is, each proband was given point values considering the direction of avoiding circular logic and combined values, and then the strength level for PM3 was determined. For the PP3 criterion, REVEL (>0.75 for missense variants) [12,13], MutationTaster [14], MaxEntScan (for predicted impact on splicing) [15], and spliceAI (for the predicted impact on splicing) [16] were used. For checking critical functional domains (catalytic barrel and active site) when applying the PVS1 ACMG/AMP variant criterion, Pfam (https://pfam.xfam.org/, accessed on 20 March 2021), InterPro (https://www.ebi.ac.uk/interpro/, accessed on 20 March 2021), and UniProt (https://www.uniprot.org/, accessed on 20 March 2021) were used. Among the *GAA* variants reported in the Pompe disease *GAA* variant database, variants reported as pathogenic or likely pathogenic variants (PLPVs) with a review status of ≥2 gold stars in ClinVar (https://www.ncbi.nlm.nih.gov/clinvar/, assessed on 27 April 2021) were classified as *GAA* PLPVs.

2.3. Analysis of Carrier Frequency and Predicted Genetic Prevalence

The carrier frequency (CF) and predicted genetic prevalence (pGP) were analyzed based on the heterozygous PLPVs. Neither the KRGDB nor the jMorp database provides information about homozygous variants. Thus (likely) pathogenic variants found in these databases were considered heterozygous variants because the general population assumes that there are no rare diseases. The CF and pGP were calculated as previously described [8,17].

3. Results

3.1. GAA Variants Found in Patients with Pompe Disease or General Population Databases

The *GAA* variants in Korean or Japanese patients with Pompe disease reported in previous studies are described in Table 1. A total of 10 studies evaluating the *GAA* variants in Korean patients with Pompe disease were reviewed [18–27]. To date, 17 different PLPVs (total of 59 PLPV alleles) in *GAA* have been reported in 32 Korean patients with Pompe disease (Table 1). *GAA* variants classified as variants of uncertain significance (VUS) because of insufficient pathogenic evidence (c.1669A>T (p.Ile557Phe) and c.2132C>G (p.Thr711Arg) reported by Kim EH et al. [27]) or *GAA* variants described in an incorrect nomenclature were excluded in this study. A total of 17 studies on Japanese patients with Pompe disease were reviewed [28–44], and 29 different *GAA* PLPVs (total of 130 PLPV alleles) were reported in 76 Japanese patients with Pompe disease. Of the *GAA* variants reported in 17 Japanese studies, 11 were classified as VUS and one was classified as benign, which were excluded from this analysis.

Table 1. Pathogenic or likely pathogenic variants found in Korean or Japanese patients with Pompe disease or in general population databases.

Variant	Korean Patients		Japanese Patients		General Population Databases, MAF			
	Allele Count	[Ref] (HT/HM)	Allele Count	[Ref] (HT/HM)	KRGDB [1]	jMorp [2]	gnomAD [3], East Asian	gnomAD [3], Global
c.-32-13T>G	0		0		0.000342	0	0.000207	0.003401
c.2T>C	0		1	[28] (1/0)	0	0	0	0
c.118C>T (p.Arg40 *)	1	[20] (1/0)	1	[28] (1/0)	0	0	0.000050	0.000014
c.169C>T (p.Gln57 *)	0		1	[28] (1/0)	0	0	0	0
c.307T>C (p.Cys103Arg)	0		0		0	0.000060	0	0
c.309C>A (p.Cys103 *)	0		2	[29] (0/1)	0	0	0	0
c.483dup (p.Lys162Glnfs*15)	0		2	[30] (2/0)	0	0	0	0
c.546G>A (p.Thr182=)	0		0		0	0.000179	0.000102	0.000030
c.546G>T (p.Thr182=)	2	[22] (1/0), [25] (1/0)	27	[28] (6/5), [34] (0/2), [35] (2/1), [36] (1/0), [37] (0/1)	0	0.000119	0	0
c.547-1G>C	0		1	[28] (1/0)	0	0	0	0
c.569G>A (p.Arg190His)	0		1	[28] (1/0)	0	0.000060	0	0.000016
c.655G>A (p.Gly219Arg)	0		1	[28] (1/0)	0	0	0	0.000018
c.670C>T (p.Arg224Trp)	0		1	[31] (1/0)	0	0	0	0.000022
(c.752C>T; c.761C>T) ((p.Ser251Leu; p.Ser254Leu)	0		2	[28] (1/0)	0.005476	0.001850	0.002759	0.000195
c.756_757insT (p.Pro253Serfs*77)	0		1	[28] (1/0)	0	0	0	0
c.796C>T (p.Pro266Ser)	1	[26] (1/0)	2	[28] (2/0)	0	0	0	0
c.841C>T (p.Arg281Trp)	0		0		0	0.000060	0	0.000205
c.875A>G (p.Tyr292Cys)	4	[18] (1/0), [19] (1/0), [21] (1/0), [23] (1/0)	0		0	0	0	0.000008
c.1156C>T (p.Gln386 *)	1	[23] (1/0)	0		0	0	0	0
c.1225dup (p.Asp409Glyfs*97)	1	[20] (1/0)	0		0	0	0	0
c.1309C>T (p.Arg437Cys)	3	[18] (1/0), [19] (1/0), [25] (1/0)	12	[28] (6/0), [33] (2/0), [38] (1/0), [39] (0/1), [40] (1/0)	0	0.000060	0	0.000008
c.1316T>A (p.Met439Lys)	14	[18] (4/0), [19] (1/0), [20] (1/0), [22] (1/0), [23] (1/0), [24] (1/0), [25] (3/0), [26] (2/0)	3	[28] (0/1), [35] (1/0)	0.001027	0	0.000384	0.000028
c.1322_1326+9del	2	[18] (1/0), [19] (1/0)	0		0	0	0	0
c.1447G>A (p.Gly483Arg)	0		0		0	0.000060	0	0.000008
c.1579_1580del (p.Arg527Glyfs*3)	2	[19] (1/0), [20] (1/0)	0		0	0	0	0.000004
c.1582_1583del (p.Gly528Leufs*2)	1	[18] (1/0)	0		0	0	0	0
c.1585_1586delinsGT (p.Ser529Val)	0		7	[32] (2/2), [41] (1/0)	0	0	0	0
c.1696T>C (p.Ser566Pro)	0		4	[28] (2/0), [30] (2/0)	0	0	0	0
c.1735G>A (p.Glu579Lys)	0		2	[28] (1/0), [42] (1/0)	0	0	0	0.000007
c.1798C>T (p.Arg600Cys)	0		20	[28] (7/0), [31] (1/0), [32] (7/1), [35] (2/0), [36] (1/0)	0	0.000239	0	0.000004
c.1822C>T (p.Arg608 *)	6	[18] (2/0), [19] (2/0), [22] (1/0), [24] (1/0)	4	[28] (1/1), [35] (1/0)	0	0	0.000051	0.000018
c.1826dup (p.Tyr609 *)	0		1	[28] (1/0)	0	0	0	0.000008
c.1857C>G (p.Ser619Arg)	7	[20] (1/0), [21] (1/0), [23] (2/0), [24] (1/0), [25] (1/0), [26] (1/0)	15	[28] (4/3), [31] (0/1), [33] (0/1), [42] (1/0)	0.000342	0.000418	0	0
c.1935C>A (p.Asp645Glu)	0		3	[32] (1/1)	0	0	0.001729	0.000124

Table 1. Cont.

Variant	Korean Patients		Japanese Patients		General Population Databases, MAF			
	Allele Count	[Ref] (HT/HM)	Allele Count	[Ref] (HT/HM)	KRGDB [1]	jMorp [2]	gnomAD [3], East Asian	gnomAD [3], Global
c.1979G>A (p.Arg660His)	0		2	[31] (2/0)	0	0	0	0.000037
c.2014C>T (p.Arg672Trp)	0		0		0	0.000060	0	0.000008
c.2015G>A (p.Arg672Gln)	5	[20] (1/0), [24] (2/0), [25] (1/0), [26] (1/0)	8	[32] (2/2), [43] (0/1)	0.000343	0	0.000111	0.000021
c.2171C>A (p.Ala724Asp)	3	[18] (1/0), [19] (1/0), [25] (1/0)	0		0	0	0	0
c.2177C>G (p.Pro726Arg)	0		2	[28] (1/0), [40] (1/0)	0	0	0	0
c.2297A>G (p.Tyr766Cys)	0		1	[28] (1/0)	0	0	0	0.000025
c.2238G>C (p.Trp746Cys)	5	[19] (1/0), [22] (1/0), [24] (1/0), [25] (2/0)	0		0.000685	0	0.000351	0.000308
c.2238G>T (p.Trp746Cys)	0		0		0	0.000119	0	0
c.2326C>T (p.Gln776 *)	0		2	[33] (2/0)	0	0	0	0
c.2407_2413del (p.Gln803 *)	1	[23] (1/0)	0		0	0	0	0
c.2481+1G>A	0		1	[28] (1/0)	0	0	0	0
c.2647-7G>A	0		0		0.000342	0.000298	0	0.000018

[1] The Korean Reference Genome Database (KRGDB, http://coda.nih.go.kr/coda/KRGDB/index.jsp, accessed on 8 February 2021). [2] The Japanese Multi Omics Reference Panel (jMorp, https://jmorp.megabank.tohoku.ac.jp/202102/variants, accessed on 16 March 2021). [3] The Genome Aggregation Database (gnomAD, https://gnomad.broadinstitute.org/, accessed on 17 March 2021). *, stop codon; Ref, references; HT, heterozygous allele count; HM, homozygous allele count; MAF, minor allele frequency.

There were 277 *GAA* variants with MAF < 1% in KRGDB, 587 variants in jMorp, and 470 variants in the East Asian population in gnomAD (Figure 2a). Of those, 47 variants were included in three databases. In addition, there were 7 *GAA* PLPVs in KRGDB and 13 PLPVs in jMorp (1 suspicious PLPV (>100 bp indel) was excluded) (Table 1, Figure 2b). Most of the (likely) pathogenic variants (with a review status of ≥ 2 gold stars in ClinVar) reported in the Pompe disease *GAA* variant database were not found in East Asian general population databases, such as KRGDB, JMorp, and gnomAD East Asian (81.6% (120/147), Figure 2a).

Overall, a total of 46 different variants from previous Korean or Japanese studies, KRGDB, or jMorp were classified into PLPVs (Table 1). Of those, 4 PLPVs were in both Korean patients and KRGDB, 6 PLPVs were in both Japanese patients and jMorp, and only 1 PLPV (c.1857C>G, p.Ser619Arg) was found in all Korean and Japanese patients, KRGDB, and jMorp (Figure 2b). Of the 46 PLPVs, there were 21 (likely) pathogenic variants with a review status of 2 or more gold stars (2 or 3) in ClinVar (https://www.ncbi.nlm.nih.gov/clinvar/, assessed on 27 April 2021), and the other 25 were (likely) pathogenic variants with a review status of <2 gold stars (0 or 1), variants of uncertain significance, variants with conflicting interpretations of pathogenicity, or absent in ClinVar. The ACMG evidence codes for the other 25 variants are described in Table S1.

Of the 900 *GAA* variants reported in the Pompe disease *GAA* variant database, 147 variants were classified as PLPVs with a review status of ≥ 2 gold stars in ClinVar (https://www.ncbi.nlm.nih.gov/clinvar/, assessed on 27 April 2021) (Figure 2c). Among those, 80 PLPVs were found in gnomAD.

3.2. Correlation between Patients with Pompe Disease and Unaffected Carriers

It was found that the overall distribution of clinical severity associated with *GAA* PLPVs detected in patients with Pompe disease and those in unaffected carriers differed (Figure 3). Especially, more *GAA* PLPVs associated with classic infantile Pompe disease were found in patients with Pompe disease than in unaffected carriers.

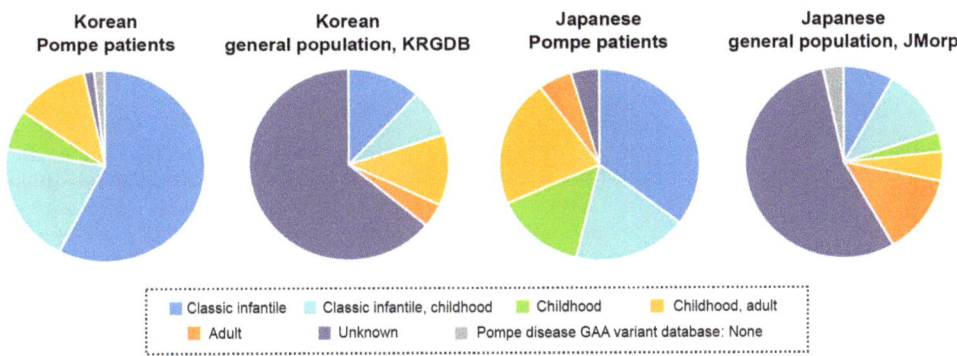

Figure 3. Overall distribution of clinical severity associated with *GAA* (likely) pathogenic variants detected in Korean or Japanese patients with Pompe disease and those found in unaffected carriers.

Spearman's correlation coefficient between the proportion of certain PLPVs among all PLPVs found in total Korean patients (for simplicity, the proportion of certain PLPVs) and the MAF of their variants in KRGDB was 0.69 ($p = 0.002$), and it was 0.45 ($p = 0.014$) for Japanese patients. In addition, Spearman's correlation coefficient between the proportion of certain PLPVs in the Pompe disease *GAA* variant database and their MAF in gnomAD (global) was 0.54 ($p = 2.64 \times 10^{-12}$) (Figure 4a).

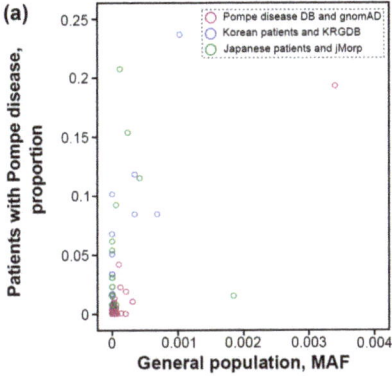
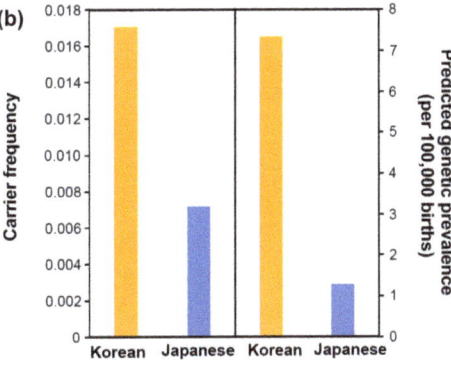

Figure 4. (**a**) Scatterplot of the proportion of certain (likely) pathogenic variants among all (likely) pathogenic variants found in total patients considering the frequency of detection (Y) and the minor allele frequency of those variants in a general population database (X). Purple line circles for patients found in the Pompe disease *GAA* variant database (Pompe disease DB), blue line circles for Korean patients, and green line circles for Japanese patients; (**b**) carrier frequency and predicted genetic prevalence for Pompe disease in Koreans and Japanese.

3.3. Carrier Frequency and Predicted Genetic Prevalence Based on General Population Databases

The total CF for Pompe disease in Koreans was estimated to be 1.7%, and the pGP was 1:13,657 (7.32 per 100,000 births) based on KRGDB (Figure 4b). In addition, the CF for Pompe disease in Japanese was predicted to be 0.7%, and the pGP was 1:78,013 (1.28 per 100,000 births) based on jMorp (Figure 4b).

4. Discussion

The main questions in this study are how *GAA* variants detected in Pompe patients are related to those in unaffected carriers and, on the contrary, how genomic information from the healthy population reflects the likelihood of developing Pompe disease. Two aspects can be considered to analyze how much *GAA* PLPVs found in patients and unaffected carriers have in common. One is to consider the qualitative aspect and to analyze how identical the *GAA* PLPVs between two groups are. The other is the quantitative aspect, which is whether certain *GAA* PLPVs frequently found in patients with Pompe disease are also found at a high frequency in unaffected carriers. In this study, Koreans and Japanese and a wider range of ethnic groups were independently analyzed to identify questions related to Pompe disease and associated *GAA* variants.

Of the 17 different PLPVs detected in Korean patients with Pompe disease, 23.5% (4 PLPVs) were found in unaffected Korean carriers in KRGDB. In addition, 20.7% (6/29) of the PLPVs detected in Japanese patients were found in unaffected Japanese carriers in JMorp (Figure 2b and Table 1). Among the PLPVs detected in Korean or Japanese patients with Pompe disease, certain PLPVs were not found in any general population databases, such as KRGDB, jMorp, and gnomAD (e.g., c.796C>T (p.Pro266Ser), c.2171C>A (p.Ala724Asp), c.1585_1586delinsGT (p.Ser529Val), c.1696T>C (p.Ser566Pro)). This means that there are *GAA* variants that are enriched especially in patients, which contribute to the development of Pompe disease. In contrast, about 50% of the PLPVs in unaffected carriers are also found in real patients with Pompe disease (Koreans, 57.1%; Japanese, 46.2%) (Figure 2b). When considering *GAA* PLPVs found in both patients and unaffected carriers, the sum of the proportion of these PLPVs (among all PLPVs found in total patients) in patients occupied up to 50%–60% (52.5% in Korean patients and 59.2% in Japanese patients).

In addition, there was a moderate positive correlation (Spearman's correlation coefficient of 0.45–0.69) between the proportion of certain PLPVs in patients and the MAF of their variants in a general population database in each of the three independent analyses. However, not all cases where PLPVs were detected in patients with Pompe disease are reported in the literature, so there is a limit to the accuracy of the proportion of certain PLPVs. In this study, Koreans were predicted to have higher CF and pGP than Japanese, and what is interesting is that Spearman's correlation coefficient in Koreans (0.69) is also higher than in Japanese (0.45).

The incidence of Pompe disease has been estimated to be 1 in 40,000, but varies depending on the geographic region or population [1]. However, the incidence of Pompe disease reported by the NBS is much higher than the estimate [4,8]. Pompe disease has not yet been included in the Korean NBS program. It is important to estimate the incidence or prevalence rate of a disease when considering its inclusion in the newborn screening program. To date, the prevalence or incidence of Pompe disease in Koreans has not been studied. The pGP (1:13,657, 7.32 per 100,000 births) for Korean Pompe disease in this study is comparable to the incidence of 1:16,919 from an NBS program involving 473,738 newborn samples in Taiwan [45]. In this study, the pGP for Pompe disease in Japanese was 1:78,013 (1.28 per 100,000 births). According to a recent study of 103,204 newborns in Japan, the incidence of Pompe disease in Japanese is 1:34,401 (three patients with potential LOPD were identified) [46]. In these three newborns, [c.752C>T; c.761C>T] ([p.Ser251Leu; p.Ser254Leu]) variant was commonly detected, and additionally, c.317G>A (p.Arg106His), c.2003A>G (p.Tyr668Cys), and c.1244C>T (p.Thr415Met) were detected, respectively. According to the 2015 ACMG/AMP guidelines [11] and specifications by a ClinGen lysosomal storage disorders expert panel (https://clinicalgenome.org/affiliation/50009/, accessed on 20 March 2021), the additional three *GAA* variants are classified as VUS. Therefore, if *GAA* variants are classified according to the current guidelines and specifications, the incidence of Pompe disease in Japanese might be lower than 1:34,401.

Interestingly, there were differences in the distribution of PLPVs detected in East Asia. The c.1316T>A (p.Met439Lys) variant was the most frequently detected in Korean patients and the second most frequent in the Korean general population, but was not found in other populations in gnomAD. This variant is supposed to be a founder pathogenic variant for Korean Pompe disease. In addition, c.546G>T (p.Thr182=) was the most reported variant in Japanese patients, and none other than the Japanese general population was reported. In addition, c.1316T>A (p.Met439Lys) and c.546G>T (p.Thr182=) were only reported in Korean or Japanese patients in the Pompe disease *GAA* variant database [9] (http://www.pompevariantdatabase.nl/, last accessed on 27 April 2021). The (c.752C>T; c.761C>T) (p.Ser251Leu; p.Ser254Leu) variant has the highest AF in both KRGDB and jMorp. However, this variant was not identified in Korean patients with Pompe disease and was identified in only one Japanese patient with a homozygous status [28]. This variant has been reported as a common causative variant in Asia, but is mostly identified on the NBS (http://www.pompevariantdatabase.nl/ accessed on 27 April 2021). It is presumed that the clinical severity associated with this variant might be very mild. Therefore, Pompe disease with this variant could not be identified. Additionally, the haplotype frequency (including this variant) for developing Pompe disease might be extremely rare. The c.-32-13T>G variant is the most common pathogenic variant for European Pompe disease [1]. However, this variant was only found in KRGDB and not reported in any Korean or Japanese patients with Pompe disease. The c.2238G>C (p.Trp746Cys) variant was reported as a common pathogenic variant for Pompe disease in mainland China [2]; however, this variant has not been reported in Japanese patients.

5. Conclusions

In this study, two different approaches were made to study Pompe disease. One was to analyze *GAA* variants based on patients in a traditional way, and the other was to analyze how likely this disease was in the general population. To apply this analysis, the *GAA* variants found in patients and the general population were interpreted as the same criterion according to the standards/guidelines or specifications for the interpretation of genetic variants, and Pompe disease in Koreans and Japanese was analyzed as a model. In addition, *GAA* PLPVs (with a review status of ≥2 gold stars in ClinVar) in the Pompe disease *GAA* variant database and gnomAD were compared.

Although some real PLPVs may have been classified as VUS due to currently insufficient evidence and the accuracy of this analysis is limited because *GAA* variants in patients with Pompe disease have been analyzed in only those reported in previous studies, the relationship between *GAA* variants found in patients with Pompe disease and in the general population is predicted to be more than a moderate correlation.

Supplementary Materials: The following are available online at https://www.mdpi.com/article/10.3390/children8070601/s1: Table S1: Presumed pathogenic or likely pathogenic variants in the *GAA* gene are found in Korean or Japanese patients or in general population databases.

Funding: This research received no external funding.

Institutional Review Board Statement: Not applicable.

Informed Consent Statement: Not applicable.

Data Availability Statement: All data analyzed in this study are included in this article and its Supplementary Information files.

Acknowledgments: The author thanks Jong-Won Kim at the Department of Laboratory Medicine and Genetics, Samsung Medical Center, Sungkyunkwan University School of Medicine, for his valuable comments on this research.

Conflicts of Interest: The author declares no conflict of interest.

References

1. van der Ploeg, A.T.; Reuser, A.J. Pompe's disease. *Lancet* **2008**, *372*, 1342–1353. [CrossRef]
2. Peruzzo, P.; Pavan, E.; Dardis, A. Molecular genetics of Pompe disease: A comprehensive overview. *Ann. Transl. Med.* **2019**, *7*, 278. [CrossRef]

3. Gungor, D.; Reuser, A.J. How to describe the clinical spectrum in Pompe disease? *Am. J. Med. Genet. A* **2013**, *161A*, 399–400. [CrossRef] [PubMed]
4. Bodamer, O.A.; Scott, C.R.; Giugliani, R.; Pompe Disease Newborn Screening Working, G. Newborn Screening for Pompe Disease. *Pediatrics* **2017**, *140*, S4–S13. [CrossRef]
5. Jung, K.S.; Hong, K.W.; Jo, H.Y.; Choi, J.; Ban, H.J.; Cho, S.B.; Chung, M. KRGDB: The large-scale variant database of 1722 Koreans based on whole genome sequencing. *Database* **2020**, *2020*. [CrossRef] [PubMed]
6. Tadaka, S.; Saigusa, D.; Motoike, I.N.; Inoue, J.; Aoki, Y.; Shirota, M.; Koshiba, S.; Yamamoto, M.; Kinoshita, K. jMorp: Japanese Multi Omics Reference Panel. *Nucleic Acids Res.* **2018**, *46*, D551–D557. [CrossRef]
7. Tadaka, S.; Hishinuma, E.; Komaki, S.; Motoike, I.N.; Kawashima, J.; Saigusa, D.; Inoue, J.; Takayama, J.; Okamura, Y.; Aoki, Y.; et al. jMorp updates in 2020: Large enhancement of multi-omics data resources on the general Japanese population. *Nucleic Acids Res.* **2021**, *49*, D536–D544. [CrossRef]
8. Park, K.S. Carrier frequency and predicted genetic prevalence of Pompe disease based on a general population database. *Mol. Genet. Metab. Rep.* **2021**, *27*, 100734. [CrossRef]
9. Nino, M.Y.; In 't Groen, S.L.M.; Bergsma, A.J.; van der Beek, N.; Kroos, M.; Hoogeveen-Westerveld, M.; van der Ploeg, A.T.; Pijnappel, W. Extension of the Pompe mutation database by linking disease-associated variants to clinical severity. *Hum. Mutat.* **2019**, *40*, 1954–1967. [CrossRef] [PubMed]
10. Heberle, H.; Meirelles, G.V.; da Silva, F.R.; Telles, G.P.; Minghim, R. InteractiVenn: A web-based tool for the analysis of sets through Venn diagrams. *BMC Bioinform.* **2015**, *16*, 169. [CrossRef]
11. Richards, S.; Aziz, N.; Bale, S.; Bick, D.; Das, S.; Gastier-Foster, J.; Grody, W.W.; Hegde, M.; Lyon, E.; Spector, E.; et al. Standards and guidelines for the interpretation of sequence variants: A joint consensus recommendation of the American College of Medical Genetics and Genomics and the Association for Molecular Pathology. *Genet. Med.* **2015**, *17*, 405–424. [CrossRef] [PubMed]
12. Ioannidis, N.M.; Rothstein, J.H.; Pejaver, V.; Middha, S.; McDonnell, S.K.; Baheti, S.; Musolf, A.; Li, Q.; Holzinger, E.; Karyadi, D.; et al. REVEL: An Ensemble Method for Predicting the Pathogenicity of Rare Missense Variants. *Am. J. Hum. Genet.* **2016**, *99*, 877–885. [CrossRef] [PubMed]
13. Ghosh, R.; Oak, N.; Plon, S.E. Evaluation of in silico algorithms for use with ACMG/AMP clinical variant interpretation guidelines. *Genome Biol.* **2017**, *18*, 225. [CrossRef] [PubMed]
14. Schwarz, J.M.; Cooper, D.N.; Schuelke, M.; Seelow, D. MutationTaster2: Mutation prediction for the deep-sequencing age. *Nat. Methods* **2014**, *11*, 361–362. [CrossRef] [PubMed]
15. Yeo, G.; Burge, C.B. Maximum entropy modeling of short sequence motifs with applications to RNA splicing signals. *J. Comput. Biol.* **2004**, *11*, 377–394. [CrossRef] [PubMed]
16. Jaganathan, K.; Kyriazopoulou Panagiotopoulou, S.; McRae, J.F.; Darbandi, S.F.; Knowles, D.; Li, Y.I.; Kosmicki, J.A.; Arbelaez, J.; Cui, W.; Schwartz, G.B.; et al. Predicting Splicing from Primary Sequence with Deep Learning. *Cell* **2019**, *176*, 535–548.e524. [CrossRef] [PubMed]
17. Hanany, M.; Rivolta, C.; Sharon, D. Worldwide carrier frequency and genetic prevalence of autosomal recessive inherited retinal diseases. *Proc. Natl. Acad. Sci. USA* **2020**, *117*, 2710–2716. [CrossRef]
18. Cho, A.; Kim, S.J.; Lim, B.C.; Hwang, H.; Park, J.D.; Kim, G.B.; Jin, D.K.; Lee, J.; Ki, C.S.; Kim, K.J.; et al. Infantile Pompe disease: Clinical and genetic characteristics with an experience of enzyme replacement therapy. *J. Child Neurol.* **2012**, *27*, 319–324. [CrossRef]
19. Kim, M.S.; Song, A.; Im, M.; Huh, J.; Kang, I.S.; Song, J.; Yang, A.; Kim, J.; Kwon, E.K.; Choi, E.J.; et al. Clinical and molecular characterization of Korean children with infantile and late-onset Pompe disease: 10 years of experience with enzyme replacement therapy at a single center. *Korean J. Pediatr.* **2019**, *62*, 224–234. [CrossRef]
20. Ko, J.M.; Park, K.S.; Kang, Y.; Nam, S.H.; Kim, Y.; Park, I.; Chae, H.W.; Lee, S.M.; Lee, K.A.; Kim, J.W. A New Integrated Newborn Screening Workflow Can Provide a Shortcut to Differential Diagnosis and Confirmation of Inherited Metabolic Diseases. *Yonsei Med. J.* **2018**, *59*, 652–661. [CrossRef]
21. Lee, D.H.; Qiu, W.J.; Lee, J.; Chien, Y.H.; Hwu, W.L. Hypertrophic cardiomyopathy in pompe disease is not limited to the classic infantile onset phenotype. *JIMD Rep.* **2014**, *17*, 71–75. [CrossRef]
22. Lee, J.H.; Shin, J.H.; Park, H.J.; Kim, S.Z.; Jeon, Y.M.; Kim, H.K.; Kim, D.S.; Choi, Y.C. Targeted population screening of late onset Pompe disease in unspecified myopathy patients for Korean population. *Neuromuscul. Disord.* **2017**, *27*, 550–556. [CrossRef]
23. Park, H.D.; Lee, D.H.; Choi, T.Y.; Lee, Y.K.; Lee, S.Y.; Kim, J.W.; Ki, C.S.; Lee, Y.W. Three patients with glycogen storage disease type II and the mutational spectrum of GAA in Korean patients. *Ann. Clin. Lab. Sci.* **2013**, *43*, 311–316. [PubMed]
24. Park, H.J.; Jang, H.; Kim, J.H.; Lee, J.H.; Shin, H.Y.; Kim, S.M.; Park, K.D.; Yim, S.V.; Lee, J.H.; Choi, Y.C. Discovery of pathogenic variants in a large Korean cohort of inherited muscular disorders. *Clin. Genet.* **2017**, *91*, 403–410. [CrossRef]
25. Park, J.S.; Kim, H.G.; Shin, J.H.; Choi, Y.C.; Kim, D.S. Effect of enzyme replacement therapy in late onset Pompe disease: Open pilot study of 48 weeks follow-up. *Neurol. Sci.* **2015**, *36*, 599–605. [CrossRef] [PubMed]
26. Park, Y.E.; Park, K.H.; Lee, C.H.; Kim, C.M.; Kim, D.S. Two new missense mutations of GAA in late onset glycogen storage disease type II. *J. Neurol. Sci.* **2006**, *251*, 113–117. [CrossRef]
27. Kim, E.H.; Ko, J.M.; Lee, B.H.; Kim, G.H.; Choi, J.H.; Yoo, H.W. Two patients with atypical infantile Pompe disesase presenting with hypertrophic cardiomyopathy. *J. Genet. Med.* **2009**, *6*, 161–165.

28. Fukuhara, Y.; Fuji, N.; Yamazaki, N.; Hirakiyama, A.; Kamioka, T.; Seo, J.H.; Mashima, R.; Kosuga, M.; Okuyama, T. A molecular analysis of the GAA gene and clinical spectrum in 38 patients with Pompe disease in Japan. *Mol. Genet. Metab. Rep.* **2018**, *14*, 3–9. [CrossRef]
29. Hermans, M.M.; van Leenen, D.; Kroos, M.A.; Beesley, C.E.; Van Der Ploeg, A.T.; Sakuraba, H.; Wevers, R.; Kleijer, W.; Michelakakis, H.; Kirk, E.P.; et al. Twenty-two novel mutations in the lysosomal alpha-glucosidase gene (GAA) underscore the genotype-phenotype correlation in glycogen storage disease type II. *Hum. Mutat.* **2004**, *23*, 47–56. [CrossRef] [PubMed]
30. Matsuoka, T.; Miwa, Y.; Tajika, M.; Sawada, M.; Fujimaki, K.; Soga, T.; Tomita, H.; Uemura, S.; Nishino, I.; Fukuda, T.; et al. Divergent clinical outcomes of alpha-glucosidase enzyme replacement therapy in two siblings with infantile-onset Pompe disease treated in the symptomatic or pre-symptomatic state. *Mol. Genet. Metab. Rep.* **2016**, *9*, 98–105. [CrossRef]
31. Pipo, J.R.; Feng, J.H.; Yamamoto, T.; Ohsaki, Y.; Nanba, E.; Tsujino, S.; Sakuragawa, N.; Martiniuk, F.; Ninomiya, H.; Oka, A.; et al. New GAA mutations in Japanese patients with GSDII (Pompe disease). *Pediatr. Neurol.* **2003**, *29*, 284–287. [CrossRef]
32. Tsujino, S.; Huie, M.; Kanazawa, N.; Sugie, H.; Goto, Y.; Kawai, M.; Nonaka, I.; Hirschhorn, R.; Sakuragawa, N. Frequent mutations in Japanese patients with acid maltase deficiency. *Neuromuscul. Disord.* **2000**, *10*, 599–603. [CrossRef]
33. Nabatame, S.; Taniike, M.; Sakai, N.; Kato-Nishimura, K.; Mohri, I.; Kagitani-Shimono, K.; Okinaga, T.; Tachibana, N.; Ozono, K. Sleep disordered breathing in childhood-onset acid maltase deficiency. *Brain Dev.* **2009**, *31*, 234–239. [CrossRef] [PubMed]
34. Tsuburaya, R.S.; Monma, K.; Oya, Y.; Nakayama, T.; Fukuda, T.; Sugie, H.; Hayashi, Y.K.; Nonaka, I.; Nishino, I. Acid phosphatase-positive globular inclusions is a good diagnostic marker for two patients with adult-onset Pompe disease lacking disease specific pathology. *Neuromuscul. Disord.* **2012**, *22*, 389–393. [CrossRef] [PubMed]
35. Kobayashi, H.; Shimada, Y.; Ikegami, M.; Kawai, T.; Sakurai, K.; Urashima, T.; Ijima, M.; Fujiwara, M.; Kaneshiro, E.; Ohashi, T.; et al. Prognostic factors for the late onset Pompe disease with enzyme replacement therapy: From our experience of 4 cases including an autopsy case. *Mol. Genet. Metab.* **2010**, *100*, 14–19. [CrossRef] [PubMed]
36. Maimaiti, M.; Takahashi, S.; Okajima, K.; Suzuki, N.; Ohinata, J.; Araki, A.; Tanaka, H.; Mukai, T.; Fujieda, K. Silent exonic mutation in the acid-alpha-glycosidase gene that causes glycogen storage disease type II by affecting mRNA splicing. *J. Hum. Genet.* **2009**, *54*, 493–496. [CrossRef] [PubMed]
37. Hossain, M.A.; Miyajima, T.; Akiyama, K.; Eto, Y. A Case of Adult-onset Pompe Disease with Cerebral Stroke and Left Ventricular Hypertrophy. *J. Stroke Cerebrovasc. Dis.* **2018**, *27*, 3046–3052. [CrossRef]
38. Fujimoto, S.; Manabe, Y.; Fujii, D.; Kozai, Y.; Matsuzono, K.; Takahashi, Y.; Narai, H.; Omori, N.; Adachi, K.; Nanba, E.; et al. A novel mutation of the GAA gene in a patient with adult-onset Pompe disease lacking a disease-specific pathology. *Intern. Med.* **2013**, *52*, 2461–2464. [CrossRef] [PubMed]
39. Isayama, R.; Shiga, K.; Seo, K.; Azuma, Y.; Araki, Y.; Hamano, A.; Takezawa, H.; Kuriyama, N.; Takezawa, N.; Mizuno, T.; et al. Sixty six-month follow-up of muscle power and respiratory function in a case with adult-type Pompe disease treated with enzyme replacement therapy. *J. Clin. Neuromuscul. Dis.* **2014**, *15*, 152–156. [CrossRef]
40. Ishigaki, K.; Yoshikawa, Y.; Kuwatsuru, R.; Oda, E.; Murakami, T.; Sato, T.; Saito, T.; Umezu, R.; Osawa, M. High-density CT of muscle and liver may allow early diagnosis of childhood-onset Pompe disease. *Brain Dev.* **2012**, *34*, 103–106. [CrossRef]
41. Tsunoda, H.; Ohshima, T.; Tohyama, J.; Sasaki, M.; Sakuragawa, N.; Martiniuk, F. Acid alpha-glucosidase deficiency: Identification and expression of a missense mutation (S529V) in a Japanese adult phenotype. *Hum. Genet.* **1996**, *97*, 496–499. [CrossRef] [PubMed]
42. Ishigaki, K.; Murakami, T.; Nakanishi, T.; Oda, E.; Sato, T.; Osawa, M. Close monitoring of initial enzyme replacement therapy in a patient with childhood-onset Pompe disease. *Brain Dev.* **2012**, *34*, 98–102. [CrossRef]
43. Huie, M.L.; Tsujino, S.; Sklower Brooks, S.; Engel, A.; Elias, E.; Bonthron, D.T.; Bessley, C.; Shanske, S.; DiMauro, S.; Goto, Y.I.; et al. Glycogen storage disease type II: Identification of four novel missense mutations (D645N, G648S, R672W, R672Q) and two insertions/deletions in the acid alpha-glucosidase locus of patients of differing phenotype. *Biochem. Biophys. Res. Commun.* **1998**, *244*, 921–927. [CrossRef]
44. Muraoka, T.; Murao, K.; Imachi, H.; Kikuchi, F.; Yoshimoto, T.; Iwama, H.; Hosokawa, H.; Nishino, I.; Fukuda, T.; Sugie, H.; et al. Novel mutations in the gene encoding acid alpha-1,4-glucosidase in a patient with late-onset glycogen storage disease type II (Pompe disease) with impaired intelligence. *Intern. Med.* **2011**, *50*, 2987–2991. [CrossRef] [PubMed]
45. Chiang, S.C.; Hwu, W.L.; Lee, N.C.; Hsu, L.W.; Chien, Y.H. Algorithm for Pompe disease newborn screening: Results from the Taiwan screening program. *Mol. Genet. Metab.* **2012**, *106*, 281–286. [CrossRef] [PubMed]
46. Momosaki, K.; Kido, J.; Yoshida, S.; Sugawara, K.; Miyamoto, T.; Inoue, T.; Okumiya, T.; Matsumoto, S.; Endo, F.; Hirose, S.; et al. Newborn screening for Pompe disease in Japan: Report and literature review of mutations in the GAA gene in Japanese and Asian patients. *J. Hum. Genet.* **2019**, *64*, 741–755. [CrossRef]

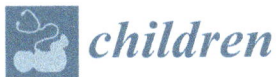

Article

Characteristics of Clinical Trial Participants with Duchenne Muscular Dystrophy: Data from the Muscular Dystrophy Surveillance, Tracking, and Research Network (MD STAR*net*)

Katherine D. Mathews [1], Kristin M. Conway [2], Amber M. Gedlinske [3], Nicholas Johnson [4], Natalie Street [5], Russell J. Butterfield [6], Man Hung [7], Emma Ciafaloni [8] and Paul A. Romitti [2,*]

1. Carver College of Medicine, The University of Iowa, Iowa City, IA 52242, USA; katherine-mathews@uiowa.edu
2. Department of Epidemiology, The University of Iowa, Iowa City, IA 52242, USA; kristin-caspers@uiowa.edu
3. Department of Internal Medicine, The University of Iowa, Iowa City, IA 52242, USA; amber-gedlinske@uiowa.edu
4. Department of Neurology, Virginia Commonwealth University, Richmond, VA 23298, USA; nicholas.johnson@vcuhealth.org
5. Centers for Disease Control and Prevention, National Center on Birth Defects and Developmental Disabilities, Atlanta, GA 30329, USA; ntl2@cdc.gov
6. Departments of Pediatrics and Neurology, University of Utah, Salt Lake City, UT 84132, USA; russell.butterfield@hsc.utah.edu
7. College of Dental Medicine, Roseman University of Health Sciences, South Jordan, UT 84095, USA; mhung@roseman.edu
8. Department of Neurology, University of Rochester, Rochester, NY 14642, USA; Emma_Ciafaloni@URMC.Rochester.edu
* Correspondence: paul-romitti@uiowa.edu; Tel.: +1-(319)-335-4912

Abstract: Background: Therapeutic trials are critical to improving outcomes for individuals diagnosed with Duchenne muscular dystrophy (DMD). Understanding predictors of clinical trial participation could maximize enrollment. Methods: Data from six sites (Colorado, Iowa, Piedmont region North Carolina, South Carolina, Utah, and western New York) of the Muscular Dystrophy Surveillance, Tracking, and Research Network (MD STAR*net*) were analyzed. Clinical trial participation and individual-level clinical and sociodemographic characteristics were obtained from medical records for the 2000–2015 calendar years. County-level characteristics were determined from linkage of the most recent county of residence identified from medical records and publicly available federal datasets. Fisher's exact and Wilcoxon two-sample tests were used with statistical significance set at one-sided *p*-value (<0.05) based on the hypothesis that nonparticipants had fewer resources. Results: Clinical trial participation was identified among 17.9% (MD STAR*net* site: 3.7–27.3%) of 358 individuals with DMD. Corticosteroids, tadalafil, and ataluren (PTC124) were the most common trial medications recorded. Fewer non-Hispanic blacks or Hispanics than non-Hispanic whites participated in clinical trials. Trial participants tended to reside in counties with lower percentages of non-Hispanic blacks. **Conclusion:** Understanding characteristics associated with clinical trial participation is critical for identifying participation barriers and generalizability of trial results. MD STAR*net* is uniquely able to track clinical trial participation through surveillance and describe patterns of participation.

Keywords: clinical trials; Duchenne muscular dystrophy; public health surveillance

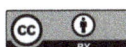

1. Introduction

The dystrophinopathies, Duchenne muscular dystrophy (DMD) and allelic Becker muscular dystrophy (BMD), are X-linked recessive disorders caused by mutations in the *DMD* gene that result in deficient dystrophin production [1]. Dystrophin is a cytoplasmic protein expressed in skeletal and cardiac muscle that links the contractile matrix to the sarcolemmal membrane, providing structural integrity during contraction. In general, DMD is associated with mutations that disrupt the reading frame or lead to a premature stop, resulting in a complete absence of dystrophin in muscle. DMD is characterized by progressive muscle weakness. Historically, males with DMD lost independent ambulation by 12 years of age and had a significantly shortened life span with death in the second or third decade of life from respiratory failure or cardiomyopathy [1–3]. Although DMD has a relatively stereotyped progression, variability is observed in the age at onset of muscle weakness and rate of progression [4]. BMD is associated with reduced or abnormal dystrophin protein and mutations that retain reading frame. BMD includes a wide spectrum of severity and is historically distinguished from DMD by having loss of independent ambulation after age 16 years.

Although advances in the multidisciplinary care, especially regarding respiratory care and use of corticosteroids, have produced considerable improvement in life expectancy [3,5–8], therapeutic trials are critical for improving outcomes in males with Duchenne muscular dystrophy (DMD) or Becker muscular dystrophy (BMD). Clinical-Trials.gov currently lists 39 interventional studies for males with DMD or BMD that are pending or actively enrolling children from birth to 17 years of age (date accessed 5 November 2021). Of these interventional studies, 24 involve some form of therapeutic drug intervention. To complete therapeutic trials as quickly as possible and have the statistical power to determine effectiveness of the therapies under study, it is desirable for all males who are eligible for therapeutic trials to have the opportunity to participate [9].

Participation in therapeutic clinical trials is often taxing on families, typically requiring missed days from work and school, travel, and long days of evaluation; thus, participation may be skewed towards those with more resources [10–13]. Further, the willingness to participate in or have access to clinical trials varies by race/ethnicity, socioeconomic status, and geographic location [14–18]. The Muscular Dystrophy Surveillance, Tracking, and Research Network (MD STAR*net*) ascertains individuals diagnosed with DMD or BMD and collects demographic and longitudinal clinical data, including clinical trial participation. Our study describes baseline associations between selected clinical and sociodemographic characteristics and participation in a therapeutic clinical trial for individuals diagnosed with Duchenne muscular dystrophy (DMD) followed by the MD STAR*net* during 2000–2015.

2. Materials and Methods

MD STAR*net* is a population-based public health surveillance program of nine muscular dystrophies, including dystrophinopathies, funded by the Centers for Disease Control and Prevention. Details about MD STAR*net* were published previously [19–24]. For this study, retrospective active surveillance data were collected by six sites: Colorado (CO), Iowa (IA), North Carolina, Piedmont region (NC), South Carolina (SC), Utah (UT), and New York's 21 western counties (wNY). Eligibility for case inclusion in this study included having data on dates of birth and diagnosis of DMD or BMD on or after 1 January 2000, residency in an MD STAR*net* surveillance region, and a confirmed health encounter during 1 January 2000–31 December 2015.

Retrospective medical record review was completed for encounters during the eligibility period using a standardized abstraction tool that documented signs and symptoms (trouble rising/Gowers' sign, trouble walking/running/jumping, frequent falling/clumsiness, inability to keep up with peers, abnormal gait, loss of motor skills, gross motor delay, or muscle weakness), ambulation status, family history, results of diagnostic testing (genetic test; muscle biopsy—immunostaining, Western blot; CK), health encounters, medical test results documenting functioning within the respiratory, cardiac and skeletal systems, medical interventions for each system, and medications prescribed.

Using abstracted signs and symptoms, clinical test results, and family histories, individuals were assigned a clinical classification by clinical review and consensus (see Figure 1) [19]. Data for all individuals, excluding those classified with possible DMD or BMD, were pooled to create an analytical dataset. We restricted our analyses to individuals classified as definite DMD (*n* = 371) as this group was genetically confirmed. We also excluded individuals ascertained by UT, but who were residents of Nevada, due to incomplete medical record access (*n* = 13). Our final sample was comprised of 358 individuals with DMD.

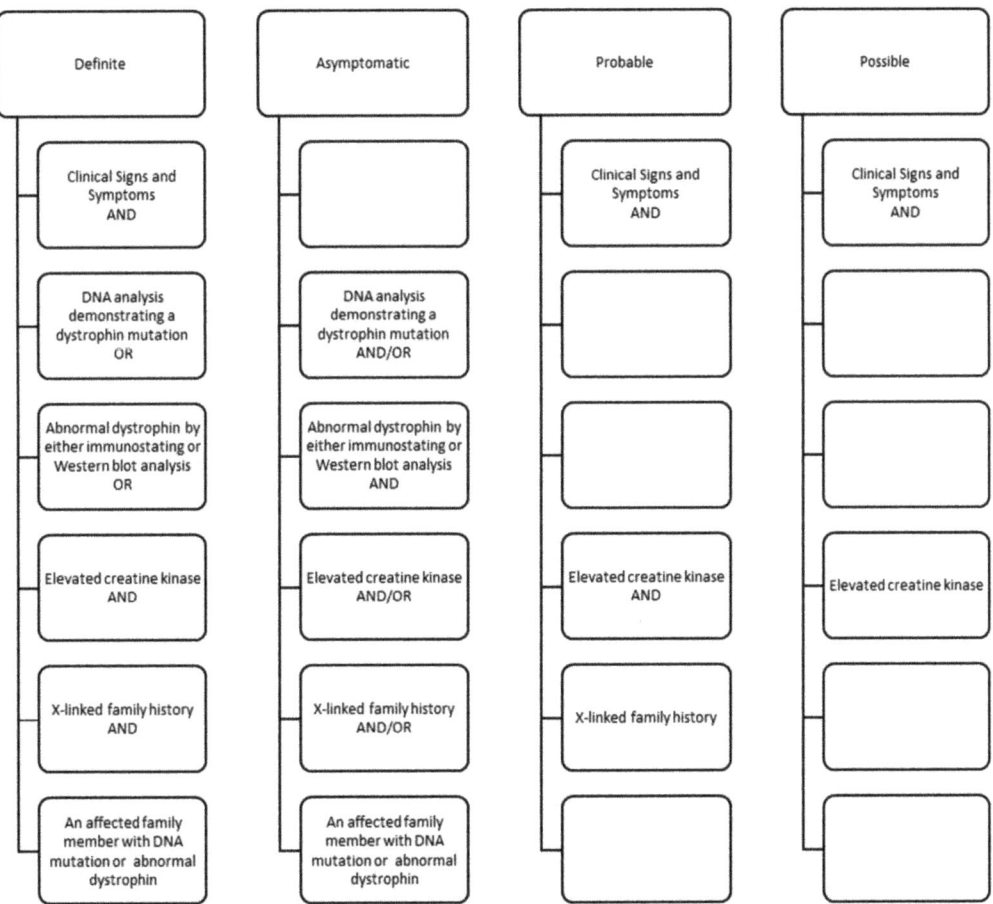

Figure 1. Clinical components for classification of males with Duchenne or Becker muscular dystrophy in the Muscular Dystrophy Surveillance, Tracking and Research Network (MD STAR*net*), 2000–2015. Classifications defined as: definite–clinical signs plus direct confirmation (pathogenic *DMD* mutation, decreased amount or size of dystrophin, or X-linked family history and elevated creatine kinase); asymptomatic–pathogenic *DMD* mutation but no clinical signs; probable–clinical signs plus elevated creatine kinase and X-linked family history; possible–clinical signs plus elevated creatine kinase, but no family history.

2.1. Clinical Trial Participation

We defined clinical trial participation based on the evidence of receiving a therapeutic non-steroidal clinical trial medication (type, year); enrollment in a corticosteroid clinical trial (year); or a checkbox for any clinical trial participation (yes/no). These indicators were combined to determine any clinical trial participation. Unless otherwise indicated, we included all individuals with any evidence of clinical trial participation. Because age at clinical trial participation was not available across all indicators of participation, we estimated the age of the individual in 2015 to describe the age distribution at the end of the surveillance period.

2.2. Clinical Characteristics

Using month and year, we estimated the age at loss of independent ambulation and classified ambulation status as walking, not walking, or unknown status. Family history of Duchenne or Becker MD was categorized as definite, suspected, no known family history, or unknown family history. Mutation type was classified as deletion, duplication, point mutation and double mutation, or unknown. Using complete dates, we calculated the age at first and last clinic visits. Finally, corticosteroid use was classified as no or yes.

2.3. Sociodemographic Characteristics

We collected race/ethnicity from the medical record for the child and from the birth certificate for the child and parents, where available. Because MD STARnet did not collect parent education and race/ethnicity from the medical record and there were limitations for linking to birth certificates for all individuals (missing ranged from 10.9–52.3% across sites), we linked the most recent county residence information collected from the medical record to publicly available national datasets that provide county-level population data for race/ethnicity, education, and economic indicators of poverty and household income. For race/ethnicity, we used population estimates for males aged 5 to 9 years in 2015 and estimated the percent of the population that was non-Hispanic white alone, non-Hispanic black alone, non-Hispanic other or combined races, and Hispanic. We used the 5-year average from the 2014–2018 American Community Survey for education and analyzed the percentage of the population that had less than a high school education, high school degree, some college, and a bachelor's degree. The 2015 economic indicators represented the median percentage of the population that met the poverty guideline and the median household income. Finally, the 2013 Rural-Urban-Continuum Codes were recategorized into the metropolitan area >1,000,000, metropolitan area 250,000–1,000,000, metropolitan area <250,000, or nonmetropolitan urban or rural adjacent to metropolitan area, and nonmetropolitan urban or rural not adjacent to metropolitan area.

2.4. Statistical Analysis

We compared percentages and mean values by clinical trial participation. Fisher's exact tests were used to test associations between categorical variables and Wilcoxon two-sample tests were used for continuous variables. Based on the hypothesis that clinical trial non-participants had fewer resources, the one-sided p-value of <0.05 was used to determine statistical significance.

3. Results

Therapeutic clinical trials for DMD active during 2000–2015 are presented in Figure 2. Overall, 17.9% of 358 individuals ascertained by the MD STARnet were identified as participating in a clinical trial (Table 1). During the period of this study, there were mutation-specific clinical trials open for patients with nonsense mutations (premature stop codons) and deletions that would have restored the reading frame by skipping exon 51.

Of all individuals, 9.5% had a mutation amenable to exon skipping treatments and 10.3% had nonsense mutations (Table 1). Of those eligible to receive a non-corticosteroid clinical trial medication, no single medication was taken by more than 15 individuals. Corticosteroids, tadalafil, and ataluren (PTC124) were the most common clinical trial medications recorded. The age of those individuals in 2015 who had participated in a clinical trial during 2000–2015 tended to cluster between 7 and 12 years (Figure 3) and most clinical trial medications were identified as having started during 2013–2015 (Figure 4).

Clinical trial participation differed by MD STARnet site, ranging from 3.7 to 27% of individuals between sites (Table 2). Individuals were identified as receiving a clinical trial medication in five sites, but participation in a corticosteroid clinical trial was only identified in two (data not shown). Clinical trial participants were more likely to be non-Hispanic white; fewer non-Hispanic blacks and Hispanics were identified as participants (Table 2). For county-level sociodemographic factors, individuals who participated in a clinical trial resided in counties with lower percentages of non-Hispanic blacks (Table 2). No statistically significant differences by clinical trial participation were found for county-level education, household income, household poverty, nor rural-urban continuum codes.

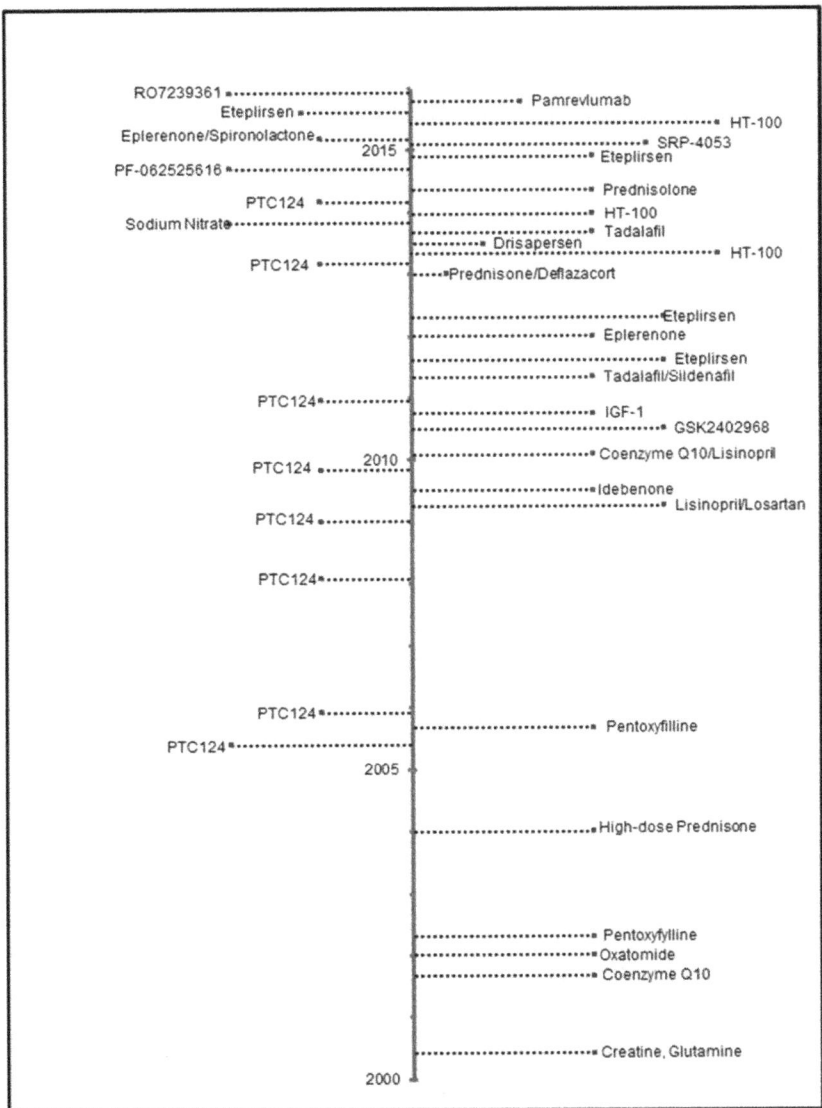

Figure 2. Dates of posting Phase 2 and 3 drug trials from ClinicalTrials.gov, using search criteria of Duchenne muscular dystrophy as disease; interventional studies as study type; and child (birth to 17 years) age. Trials were additionally limited to those occurring in the U.S. with a start date from 1 January 2000 to 31 December 2015.

Table 1. Characteristics of Clinical Trial Eligibility and Participants in the Muscular Dystrophy Surveillance, Tracking, and Research Network (MD STAR*net*), 2000–2015.

Characteristics	n (%)
Total Sample	358
Clinical Trial Eligible Mutations, All Individuals	
Exon-Skippable (exon 51) Deletions, n (% total)	34 (9.5)
Nonsense (premature stop codon) Mutations, n (% total)	37 (10.3)
Clinical Trial Participation, n (% total) [1]	64 (17.9)
Clinical Trial Checkbox	59 (16.5)
Corticosteroid Clinical Trial	15 (4.2)
Clinical Trial Medication (non-corticosteroid)	33 (9.2)
Clinical Trial Medication, n (% total medications) [2]	33
Tadalafil	9 (27.3)
Ataluren (PTC124)	9 (27.3)
Idebenone	4 (12.1)
Drisapersen (GSK2402968)	3 (9.1)
CAT-1004	2 (6.1)
IGF-1	2 (6.1)
Domegrozumab (PF-06252616)	1 (3.0)
Eplerenone	1 (3.0)
Eteplirsen	1 (3.0)
Unspecified	1 (3.0)

[1] More than one clinical trial category may be identified per individual. [2] More than one clinical trial medication may be identified per individual.

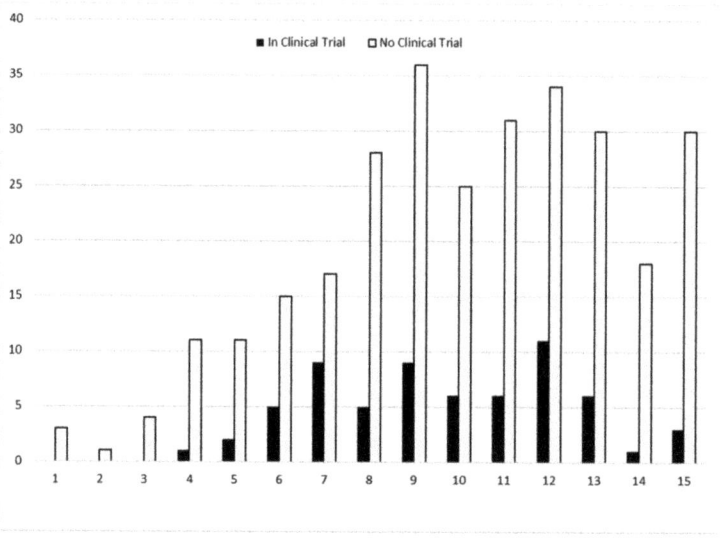

Figure 3. Number of individuals by age (years) in 2015 and clinical trial participation during 2000–2015, the Muscular Dystrophy Surveillance, Tracking, and Research Network (MD STAR*net*).

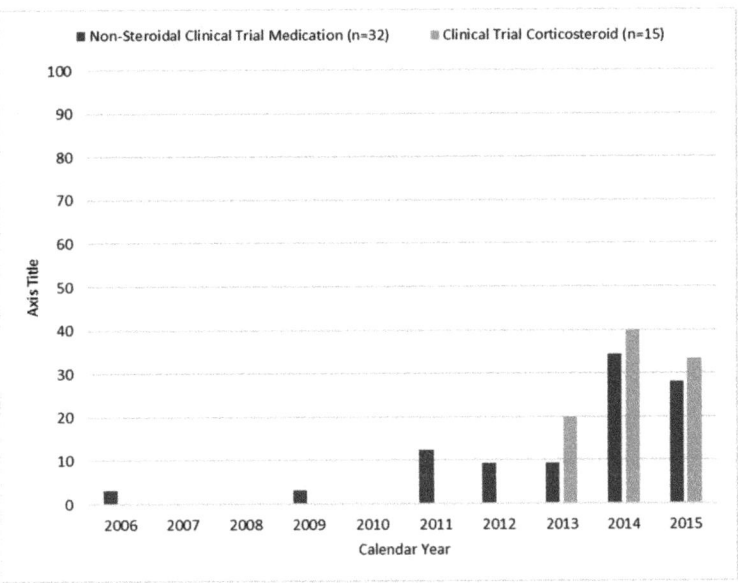

Figure 4. Frequency percentages for calendar year of initial documentation of enrollment in a clinical trial, the Muscular Dystrophy Surveillance, Tracking, and Research Network (MD STAR*net*), 2000–2015. Note: Year of use was missing for non-steroidal clinical trial medication ($n = 1$).

Table 2. Sample characteristics by any clinical trial participation in the Muscular Dystrophy Surveillance, Tracking, and Research Network (MD STAR*net*), 2000–2015.

Characteristics	In Clinical Trial	Not in Clinical Trial	*p*-Value
Total	64	294	
MD STARnet Site, *n* (row %)			0.0118 [1]
Site A	15 (17.0)	73 (83.0)	
Site B	10 (17.9)	46 (82.1)	
Site C	10 (17.0)	49 (83.0)	
Site D	12 (26.0)	34 (74.0)	
Site E	2 (3.7)	52 (96.3)	
Site F	15 (27.3)	40 (72.7)	
Child characteristics			
Child Race/Ethnicity, *n* (row %)			0.0486 [1]
non-Hispanic white	52 (21.4)	191 (78.6)	
non-Hispanic black	1 (4.0)	24 (96.0)	
non-Hispanic other	2 (15.4)	11 (84.6)	
Hispanic or Latino/Latina	7 (10.8)	58 (89.2)	
Unknown	2	10	
County-level sociodemographics			
Race/ethnicity (2015), Mean (95% CL) [3]			
non-Hispanic white alone	65.5 (61.1, 70.0)	62.4 (60.6, 64.3)	0.1019 [2]
non-Hispanic black alone	8.1 (5.5, 10.7)	11.6 (10.1, 13.1)	0.0115 [2]
non-Hispanic other or combined	7.4 (6.6, 8.1)	7.4 (7.1, 7.7)	0.4596 [2]

Table 2. Cont.

Characteristics	In Clinical Trial	Not in Clinical Trial	p-Value
Hispanic	19.0 (16.4, 21.7)	18.6 (17.2, 20.0)	0.1383 [2]
Education (2014–2018), Mean (95% CL) [4]			
Less than HS	9.6 (8.9, 10.2)	10.2 (9.8, 10.7)	0.3228 [2]
HS	26.1 (24.4, 27.9)	26.3 (25.5, 27.0)	0.4385 [2]
Some college	31.7 (30.7, 32.7)	31.5 (31.0, 31.9)	0.3416 [2]
Bachelor's degree	32.6 (30.1, 35.2)	32.0 (30.8, 33.2)	0.4536 [2]
Economic indicators [5]			
Household income (2015), median (95% CL)	$58,367 ($56,067, $60,667)	$57,148 ($55,920, $58,376)	0.1631 [2]
Poverty (2015), median percent of population (95% CL)	17.0 (15.6, 18.4)	18.0 (17.3, 18.6)	0.1115 [2]
Rural-Urban Continuum Codes, n (row %) [6]			0.4656 [1]
Metropolitan area—1 million population or more	29 (22.3)	101 (77.7)	
Metropolitan area—250,000 to 1 million population	20 (14.3)	120 (85.7)	
Metropolitan area—fewer than 250,000 population	3 (12.5)	21 (87.5)	
Nonmetropolitan urban area or rural area adjacent to metropolitan area	8 (20.5)	31 (79.5)	
Nonmetropolitan urban area or rural area not adjacent to metropolitan area	3 (15.0)	17 (85.0)	

CL = confidence limits. [1] Fisher's exact test. [2] Wilcoxon two-sample test, one-sided p-value. [3] n = 353; 5 individuals with missing county. United States Census Bureau. https://www2.census.gov/programs-surveys/popest/datasets/2010-2018/counties/asrh/cc-est2018-alldata.csv (accessed on 6 June 2021). [4] n = 353; 5 individuals with missing county. U.S. Department of Agriculture Economic Research Service. U.S. Department of Agriculture county-level datasets. https://www.ers.usda.gov/data-products/county-level-data-sets/ (accessed on 6 June 2021). [5] n = 353; 5 individuals with missing county. United States Census Bureau. https://www.census.gov/data/datasets/2015/demo/saipe/2015-state-and-county.html (accessed on 6 June 2021). [6] n = 353; 5 individuals with missing county. USDA Economic Research Service. U.S. Department of Agriculture Rural-Urban Continuum Codes. https://www.ers.usda.gov/data-products/rural-urban-continuum-codes// (accessed on 6 June 2021).

Among the clinical characteristics examined, individuals who were still walking were more likely to have enrolled in a trial and most had documented corticosteroid use unrelated to participation in a clinical trial. (Table 3). No differences by clinical trial participation were found for ages at first and last clinic visits nor family history of DMD. Although our methods do not allow us to identify mutation specific trials, 14 of 37 (37.8%) individuals with a nonsense mutation and 5 of 34 (14.7%) individuals amenable to exon skipping participated in a clinical trial during this period (data not shown).

Table 3. Clinical characteristics by any clinical trial participation in the Muscular Dystrophy Surveillance, Tracking, and Research Network (MD STARnet), 2000–2015.

Characteristics	In Clinical Trial	Not in Clinical Trial	p-Value
Total	64	294	
Ages (years), Mean (95% confidence limits)			
First visit [1]	5.1 (4.4, 5.7)	4.9 (4.5, 5.2)	0.2586 [2]
Last visit	9.6 (8.9, 10.3)	9.3 (8.9, 9.7)	0.4015 [2]
Ambulation status, n (row %)			0.0225 [3]
Not walking	11 (10.6)	93 (89.4)	
Walking	53 (20.9)	201 (79.1)	

Table 3. Cont.

Characteristics	In Clinical Trial	Not in Clinical Trial	p-Value
Non-trial corticosteroid use, n (row %)			<0.0001 [3]
No	5 (4.8)	100 (95.2)	
Yes	59 (23.3)	194 (76.7)	
Family history, n (row %)			0. 3832 [3]
Definite	18 (14.9)	103 (85.1)	
Suspected	0 (0.0)	8 (100.0)	
No known	8 (22.2)	28 (77.8)	
Unknown	38 (19.7)	155 (80.3)	

[1] Missing first visit age (n = 3). [2] Wilcoxon two-sample test, one-sided p-value. [3] Fisher's exact test.

4. Discussion

DMD clinical trial participation increased from 2013 through 2015, consistent with the increasing number of phase 2 or 3 clinical trials listed on ClinicalTrials.gov. Overall, we report nearly 18% of individuals identified by the MD STAR*net* had participated in a clinical trial, which is consistent with enrollment reported by a 2013–2016 Muscular Dystrophy Association highlight of the findings from their neuromuscular disease registry [25]. We identified variation in participation by MD STAR*net* site and by race and ethnicity, at the individual or county level.

The differences we observed across MD STAR*net* site were largely due to two sites' proximity to corticosteroid clinical trials and less than expected participation at one site that does not have an MDA clinic within their surveillance region. These observations suggest the importance of family proximity to a clinical trial site, resulting in the lower burden of travel and time away from home, and emphasize the need for geographically dispersed trial sites. Our observations are also consistent with parental reports of the clinic as an important source of information about clinical trials in general and specific clinical trial options [13]. Because clinics that care for individuals with DMD differ in resources and knowledge, there is the need for broad dissemination of information about clinical trials outside of the clinic setting, a role that patient advocacy groups have increasingly taken on [10,26].

Participation in a clinical trial is not only dependent on knowledge about the trial and willingness to enroll, but also requires meeting the inclusion/exclusion criteria for the trial of interest. Each trial has distinct entry criteria, but ambulatory males aged 7–10 years who are taking corticosteroids were historically the most common target population. This group is generally able to engage in motor function outcome measures, they have a predictable rate of change without treatment, and they are at a stage of disease when meaningful change can be detected [10]. We did not find age to be a significant factor in trial participation, but our cohort was generally 5–10 years old during the period of observation. Depending on the mechanism of action of the therapeutic agent being investigated, there might be additional limitations in participation for patients with specific mutations or types of mutations. Our description of the mutations among the clinical trial participants are consistent with the targeted clinical trials open during that time.

Of the individual characteristics examined, race/ethnicity was significantly associated with participation. Compared to non-Hispanic whites, lower participation was found among non-Hispanic blacks and Hispanics. The county-level results were partly consistent; those counties in which there was lower participation had higher percentages of non-Hispanic blacks. The observation that non-Hispanic blacks and Hispanics had a lower participation rate than non-Hispanic whites is consistent with observations in other diseases [27]. We note that although it was observed that non-Hispanic blacks have a lower prevalence of DMD than non-Hispanic whites [21,24], in this study we determined the rate of participation among identified patients, so the findings cannot be explained by this diagnostic discrepancy. Many explanations were proposed for discrepancies in trial participation by race or ethnicity [26,27]. One factor that influences the probability of a parent agreeing to enroll their child in a clinical trial is trust in the medical researchers. In a study of factors influencing adolescent's parents' trust regarding clinical trials, race, education level, and clinical trial impact on the child were the most significant predictors of parental trust [28]. In our population-based study, education level as estimated by county of residence was not associated with the likelihood of trial participation. It is of interest that of all US trials undergoing an FDA review between 1995 and 1999 (primarily adult trials), for which data on race of participants were available, the percentage of non-Hispanic black participants was nationally representative and Hispanic and other non-white racial groups were under-represented [29]. Our data add to the knowledge base that highlights the importance of efforts to ensure clinical trial participation that fully represents the affected population. Consistent and accurate information available to families and communities is one approach supported by previous research [27]. This can occur in the clinical setting with a trusted provider offering information and through the efforts of advocacy organizations.

Strengths and Limitations

The MD STAR*net* conducts population-based surveillance and includes sites throughout the United States. The systematic collection of clinical and sociodemographic data from all eligible individuals, with DMD, regardless of clinical trial participation status, allows a comprehensive characterization of both participants and nonparticipants. Further, clinical data are reviewed by a team of specialists and diagnoses are systematically confirmed. Limitations include the reliance on medical records to identify clinical trial participation. Information about clinical trial participation is largely collected outside of primary medical records and may only be identified if noted by the provider who is managing neuromuscular care of the individual. Further, data completeness may differ by the type of medical record source (tertiary care, independent clinic). MD STAR*net* retrospectively identifies and longitudinally follows eligible individuals. However, loss to follow up due to a movement out of a surveillance site or receipt of care at a source not accessible by the surveillance program may underestimate the number of trial participants.

5. Conclusions

MD STAR*net* is uniquely positioned to identify and describe those who are not clinical trial participants. Observing differences between clinical trial participants and nonparticipants is critical in helping us understand possible barriers to participation and maximize generalizability of trial results. MD STAR*net* is also able to provide population-based information that describes the proportion of the patients within the surveillance areas who are participating in trials, i.e., the degree of saturation of the target population. Our established methods for monitoring clinical trial participation through surveillance and identifying a cohort for prospectively tracking patterns of clinical trial participation provides a unique opportunity to track success of the FDA initiative to reduce disparities in clinical trial research [30].

Author Contributions: Conceptualization, K.D.M., A.M.G., K.M.C., and P.A.R.; Methodology, K.D.M., K.M.C., N.J., N.S., R.J.B., E.C., and P.A.R.; Formal analysis, K.M.C. and A.M.G.; Writing—original draft preparation, K.D.M., K.M.C.; Writing—review and editing A.M.G., N.J., N.S., R.J.B., M.H., E.C., and P.A.R.; Funding acquisition, P.A.R., K.M.C., N.J., and R.J.B. All authors have read and agreed to the published version of the manuscript.

Funding: This publication was supported by the cooperative agreements DD001126, DD001119, DD001123, DD001116, DD001117, DD001108, DD001120, DD001054 funded by the Centers for Disease Control and Prevention The findings and conclusions in this report are those of the authors and do not necessarily represent the official position of the Centers for Diseases Control and Prevention.

Institutional Review Board Statement: All sites obtained Institutional Review Board (IRB) approval or exemption. Most sites (Colorado, Iowa, North Carolina, New York, South Carolina) also had public health authority to conduct surveillance for muscular dystrophy.

Informed Consent Statement: Informed consent was waived.

Data Availability Statement: Due to privacy concerns (detailed personal information was obtained from a small number of individuals living in a defined surveillance area), data from the MD STAR*net* is not publicly available. Data used for this analysis are maintained at the Centers for Disease Control and Prevention.

Acknowledgments: We would also like to thank all M.D. STAR*net* staff past and present for their contributions.

Conflicts of Interest: Katherine Mathews receives research funding from NIH U54 NS053672 and U24 NS-107181, the Friedreich's Ataxia Research Alliance, the Centers for Disease Control and Prevention (U01 DD001248) and serves as a site PI for clinical research sponsored by PTC Therapeutics Inc, Sarepta Therapeutics Inc, Pfizer Inc, FibroGen Inc, AMO, BMS, Reata, Retrotope, and Italfarmaco. Dr. Mathews is an advisory board member for Sarepta Therapeutics Inc and Dyne Therapeutics. Dr. Nicholas Johnson has received grant funding from NINDS and NCATs (R01NS104010; R21TR003184), CDC (1U01DD001242) and the FDA (7R01FD006071). He receives royalties from the CCMDHI and the CMTHI. He receives research funds from Dyne, AveXis, CSL Behring, Vertex Pharmaceuticals, Fulcrum Therapeutics, ML Bio, Sarepta, and Acceleron Pharma. He has provided consultation for AveXis, AMO Pharma, Strongbridge BioPharma, Acceleron Pharma, Fulcrum Therapeutics, Dyne, Avidity, ML Bio, and Vertex Pharmaceuticals. Dr. Russell Butterfield has received funding via contracts for clinical trials from PTC Therapeutics, Sarepta Therapeutics, Pfizer, Biogen, Carpricor, and Catabasis. He serves on scientific advisory boards for Sarepta Therapeutics, Biogen, and Pfizer. No financial disclosures or conflicts of interest are reported by the remaining collaborators.

References

1. Mercuri, E.; Bönnemann, C.G.; Muntoni, F. Muscular dystrophies. *Lancet* **2019**, *394*, 2025–2038. [CrossRef]
2. Birnkrant, D.J.; Bushby, K.; Bann, C.; Apkon, S.D.; Blackwell, A.; Colvin, M.K.; Cripe, L.; Herron, A.R.; Kennedy, A.; Kinnett, K.; et al. Diagnosis and management of Duchenne muscular dystrophy, part 3: Primary care, emergency management, psychosocial care, and transitions of care across the lifespan. *Lancet Neurol.* **2018**, *17*, 445–455. [CrossRef]
3. Passamano, L.; Taglia, A.; Palladino, A.; Viggiano, E.; D'Ambrosio, P.; Scutifero, M.; Rosaria Cecio, M.; Torre, V.; De Luca, F.; Picillo, E.; et al. Improvement of survival in Duchenne Muscular Dystrophy: Retrospective analysis of 835 patients. *Acta Myol.* **2012**, *31*, 121–125. [PubMed]
4. Humbertclaude, V.; Hamroun, D.; Bezzou, K.; Bérard, C.; Boespflug-Tanguy, O.; Bommelaer, C.; Campana-Salort, E.; Cances, C.; Chabrol, B.; Commare, M.-C.; et al. Motor and respiratory heterogeneity in Duchenne patients: Implication for clinical trials. *Eur. J. Paediatr. Neurol.* **2012**, *16*, 149–160. [CrossRef] [PubMed]
5. Gomez-Merino, E.; Bach, J.R. Duchenne Muscular Dystrophy. *Am. J. Phys. Med. Rehabil.* **2002**, *81*, 411–415. [CrossRef]
6. Bach, J.R.; Martínez-González, D. Duchenne Muscular Dystrophy: Continuous Noninvasive Ventilatory Support Prolongs Survival. *Respir. Care* **2011**, *56*, 744–750. [CrossRef]
7. Eagle, M.; Baudouin, S.V.; Chandler, C.; Giddings, D.R.; Bullock, R.; Bushby, K. Survival in Duchenne muscular dystrophy: Improvements in life expectancy since 1967 and the impact of home nocturnal ventilation. *Neuromuscul. Disord.* **2002**, *12*, 926–929. [CrossRef]
8. Ishikawa, Y.; Miura, T.; Ishikawa, Y.; Aoyagi, T.; Ogata, H.; Hamada, S.; Minami, R. Duchenne muscular dystrophy: Survival by cardio-respiratory interventions. *Neuromuscul. Disord.* **2011**, *21*, 47–51. [CrossRef]
9. Shieh, P.B. Duchenne muscular dystrophy. *Curr. Opin. Neurol.* **2015**, *28*, 542–546. [CrossRef]
10. Franson, T.; Kinnett, K.; Cripe, T.P. Unique Burdens of Pediatric Clinical Trials in Duchenne Muscular Dystrophy, April 20–21, 2017, Bethesda, Maryland, USA. *Ther. Innov. Regul. Sci.* **2019**, *53*, 154–163. [CrossRef]
11. Hoberman, A.; Shaikh, N.; Bhatnagar, S.; Haralam, M.A.; Kearney, D.H.; Colborn, D.K.; Kienholz, M.L.; Wang, L.; Bunker, C.H.; Keren, R.; et al. Factors That Influence Parental Decisions to Participate in Clinical Research. *JAMA Pediatr.* **2013**, *167*, 561–566. [CrossRef] [PubMed]
12. Engster, S.A.; Fascetti, C.; Daw, K.; Reis, E.C. Parent Perceptions of and Preferences for Participation in Child Health Research: Results from a Pediatric Practice-Based Research Network. *J. Am. Board Fam. Med.* **2019**, *32*, 685–694. [CrossRef] [PubMed]
13. Peay, H.L.; Biesecker, B.B.; Wilfond, B.S.; Jarecki, J.; Umstead, K.L.; Escolar, D.M.; Tibben, A. Barriers and facilitators to clinical trial participation among parents of children with pediatric neuromuscular disorders. *Clin. Trials* **2018**, *15*, 139–148. [CrossRef] [PubMed]

14. Tanner, A.; Kim, S.-H.; Friedman, D.B.; Foster, C.; Bergeron, C.D. Barriers to Medical Research Participation as Perceived by Clinical Trial Investigators: Communicating with Rural and African American Communities. *J. Health Commun.* **2014**, *20*, 88–96. [CrossRef]
15. Kim, S.-H.; Tanner, A.; Friedman, D.B.; Foster, C.; Bergeron, C.D. Barriers to Clinical Trial Participation: Comparing Perceptions and Knowledge of African American and White South Carolinians. *J. Health Commun.* **2015**, *20*, 816–826. [CrossRef]
16. Kim, S.-H.; Tanner, A.; Friedman, D.B.; Foster, C.; Bergeron, C.D. Barriers to Clinical Trial Participation: A Comparison of Rural and Urban Communities in South Carolina. *J. Community Health* **2013**, *39*, 562–571. [CrossRef] [PubMed]
17. Wendler, D.; Kington, R.; Madans, J.; Van Wye, G.; Christ-Schmidt, H.; Pratt, L.A.; Brawley, O.W.; Gross, C.P.; Emanuel, E. Are Racial and Ethnic Minorities Less Willing to Participate in Health Research? *PLoS Med.* **2005**, *3*, e19. [CrossRef]
18. Vose, J.M. Minority Enrollment to Clinical Trials: Road to Increased Access. *Oncology* **2021**, *35*, 107. [CrossRef]
19. Mathews, K.D.; Cunniff, C.; Kantamneni, J.R.; Ciafaloni, E.; Miller, T.; Matthews, D.; Cwik, V.; Druschel, C.; Miller, L.; Meaney, F.J.; et al. Muscular Dystrophy Surveillance Tracking and Research Network (MD STARnet): Case Definition in Surveillance for Childhood-Onset Duchenne/Becker Muscular Dystrophy. *J. Child Neurol.* **2010**, *25*, 1098–1102. [CrossRef]
20. Miller, L.A.; Romitti, P.A.; Cunniff, C.; Druschel, C.; Mathews, K.; Meaney, F.J.; Matthews, D.; Kantamneni, J.; Feng, Z.-F.; Zemblidge, N.; et al. The muscular Dystrophy Surveillance Tracking and Research Network (MD STARnet): Surveillance methodology. *Birth Defects Res. Part A Clin. Mol. Teratol.* **2006**, *76*, 793–797. [CrossRef]
21. Romitti, P.A.; Zhu, Y.; Puzhankara, S.; James, K.A.; Nabukera, S.K.; Zamba, G.K.; Ciafaloni, E.; Cunniff, C.; Druschel, C.M.; Mathews, K.D.; et al. Prevalence of Duchenne and Becker Muscular Dystrophies in the United States. *Pediatrics* **2015**, *135*, 513–521. [CrossRef] [PubMed]
22. Do, T.N.; Street, N.; Donnelly, J.; Adams, M.M.; Cunniff, C.; Fox, D.J.; Weinert, R.O.; Oleszek, J.; Romitti, P.A.; Westfield, C.P.; et al. Muscular Dystrophy Surveillance, Tracking, and Research Network pilot: Population-based surveillance of major muscular dystrophies at four U.S. sites, 2007–2011. *Birth Defects Res.* **2018**, *110*, 1404–1411. [CrossRef]
23. Wallace, B.; Smith, K.T.; Thomas, S.; Conway, K.M.; Westfield, C.; Andrews, J.G.; Weinert, R.O.; Do, T.Q.N.; Street, N. Characterization of individuals with selected muscular dystrophies from the expanded pilot of the Muscular Dystrophy Surveillance, Tracking and Research Network (MD STARnet) in the United States. *Birth Defects Res.* **2020**, *113*, 560–569. [CrossRef]
24. Zhang, Y.; Mann, J.R.; James, K.A.; McDermott, S.; Conway, K.M.; Paramsothy, P.; Smith, T.; Cai, B.; Starnet, T.M. Duchenne and Becker Muscular Dystrophies' Prevalence in MD STARnet Surveillance Sites: An Examination of Racial and Ethnic Differences. *Neuroepidemiology* **2021**, *55*, 47–55. [CrossRef]
25. Muscular Dystrophy Association. Highlights of the MDA U.S. Neuromuscular Disease Registry (2013–2016). Available online: https://www.mda.org/sites/default/files/MDA%20Registry%20Report%20Highlights_Digital_final.pdf (accessed on 18 June 2021).
26. Heller, C.; Balls-Berry, J.E.; Nery, J.D.; Erwin, P.J.; Littleton, D.; Kim, M.; Kuo, W.P. Strategies addressing barriers to clinical trial enrollment of underrepresented populations: A systematic review. *Contemp. Clin. Trials* **2014**, *39*, 169–182. [CrossRef]
27. Bendixen, R.M.; Morgenroth, L.P.; Clinard, K.L. Engaging Participants in Rare Disease Research: A Qualitative Study of Duchenne Muscular Dystrophy. *Clin. Ther.* **2016**, *38*, 1474–1484.e2. [CrossRef]
28. Cunningham-Erves, J.; Villalta-Gil, V.; Wallston, K.A.; Boyer, A.P.; Wilkins, C.H. Racial differences in two measures of trust in biomedical research. *J. Clin. Transl. Sci.* **2019**, *3*, 113–119. [CrossRef] [PubMed]
29. Evelyn, B.; Toigo, T.; Banks, D.; Pohl, D.; Gray, K.; Robins, B.; Ernat, J. Participation of racial/ethnic groups in clinical trials and race-related labeling: A review of new molecular entities approved 1995–1999. *J. Natl. Med Assoc.* **2001**, *93*, 18S–24S. [PubMed]
30. Enhancing the Diversity of Clinical Trial Populations: Eligibility Criteria, Enrollment Practices, and Trial Designs Guidance for Industry. Available online: https://www.fda.gov/regulatory-information/search-fda-guidance-documents/enhancing-diversity-clinical-trial-populations-eligibility-criteria-enrollment-practices-and-trial (accessed on 18 June 2021).

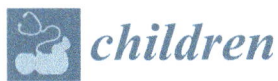

Article

Clinical Course, Myopathology and Challenge of Therapeutic Intervention in Pediatric Patients with Autoimmune-Mediated Necrotizing Myopathy

Adela Della Marina [1,*], Marc Pawlitzki [2,3], Tobias Ruck [3,4], Andreas van Baalen [5], Nadine Vogt [5], Bernd Schweiger [6], Swantje Hertel [1], Heike Kölbel [1], Heinz Wiendl [3], Corinna Preuße [7], Andreas Roos [1,8] and Ulrike Schara-Schmidt [1]

[1] Centre for Neuromuscular Disorders and Centre for Translational Neuro- and Behavioral Sciences, Department of Pediatric Neurology University Hospital Essen, University Duisburg-Essen, 45147 Essen, Germany; Swantje.Hertel@uk-essen.de (S.H.); Heike.Koelbel@uk-essen.de (H.K.); Andreas.Roos@uk-essen.de (A.R.); Ulrike.Schara-Schmidt@uk-essen.de (U.S.-S.)
[2] Department of Child and Adolescent Psychiatry and Psychotherapy, University Hospital Münster, 48149 Münster, Germany; marc.pawlitzki@ukmuenster.de
[3] Department of Neurology with Institute of Translational Neurology, University Hospital Münster, 48149 Münster, Germany; tobias.ruck@med.uni-duesseldorf.de (T.R.); heinz.wiendl@ukmuenster.de (H.W.)
[4] Department of Neurology, University Hospital Düsseldorf, Heinrich-Heine-University Düsseldorf, 40225 Düsseldorf, Germany
[5] Clinic for Child and Adolescent Medicine II, University Hospital Schleswig-Holstein, 24105 Kiel, Germany; van.baalen@pedneuro.uni-kiel.de (A.v.B.); Nadine.Vogt@uksh.de (N.V.)
[6] Institute of Diagnostic and Interventional Radiology and Neuroradiology, University Hospital Essen, University Duisburg-Essen, 45147 Essen, Germany; bernd.schweiger@uk-essen.de
[7] Department of Neuropathology, Humboldt-Universität zu Berlin and Berlin Institute of Health, Charité-Universitätsmedizin Berlin, 10117 Berlin, Germany; corinna.preusse@charite.de
[8] Children's Hospital of Eastern Ontario Research Institute, University of Ottawa, Ottawa, ON K1H 8L1, Canada
* Correspondence: Adela.Dellamarina@uk-essen.de

Abstract: (1) Background: Immune–mediated necrotizing myopathy (IMNM) is a rare form of inflammatory muscle disease which is even more rare in pediatric patients. To increase the knowledge of juvenile IMNM, we here present the clinical findings on long-term follow-up, myopathological changes, and therapeutic strategies in two juvenile patients. (2) Methods: Investigations included phenotyping, determination of antibody status, microscopy on muscle biopsies, MRI, and response to therapeutic interventions. (3) Results: Anti-signal recognition particle (anti-SRP54) and anti-3-hydroxy-3-methylglutaryl coenzyme A reductase (anti-HMGCR) antibodies (Ab) were detected in the patients. Limb girdle presentation, very high CK-levels, and a lack of skin rash at disease-manifestation and an absence of prominent inflammatory signs accompanied by an abnormal distribution of α-dystroglycan in muscle biopsies initially hinted toward a genetically caused muscle dystrophy. Further immunostaining studies revealed an increase of proteins involved in chaperone-assisted autophagy (CASA), a finding already described in adult IMNM-patients. Asymmetrical muscular weakness was present in the anti-SRP54 positive Ab patient. After initial stabilization under therapy with intravenous immunoglobulins and methotrexate, both patients experienced a worsening of their symptoms and despite further therapy escalation, developed a permanent reduction of their muscle strength and muscular atrophy. (4) Conclusions: Diagnosis of juvenile IMNM might be complicated by asymmetric muscle weakness, lack of cutaneous features, absence of prominent inflammatory changes in the biopsy, and altered α-dystroglycan.

Keywords: signal recognition particle; 3-hydroxy-3-methylglutaryl; coenzyme A reductase; juvenile myositis; therapy; clinical course; chaperone-assisted autophagy

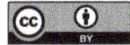

1. Introduction

Autoimmune-mediated necrotizing myopathy (IMNM) is a rare subgroup of idiopathic inflammatory myopathies (IIM) and associated with the anti-signal-recognition particle (anti-SRP54) or the anti–3-hydroxy-3-methylglutaryl-coenzyme A reductase (anti-HMGCR) autoantibodies (Ab) [1,2]. Juvenile dermatomyositis (JDM) is the most common IIM in children, with an incidence of 3.2 per million children [3], positivity for anti-HMGCR and anti-SRP54 Ab were present in only 1–2.2 % of pediatric series from the UK and the USA with IIM [1,2,4,5]. In a cohort of 387 pediatric and adult patients from Japan with IIM, 18% were anti-SRP54 and 12% were anti-HMGCR Ab positive [6], and 5% of those patients had an onset of their symptoms before 18 years of age. The presence of muscle cell necrosis and muscle cell regeneration are the histopathological hallmarks in IMNM-patient derived muscle biopsies, inflammatory cells are sparse or only slightly localized in the perivascular compartment [7,8]. Disease activity is almost always associated with elevated creatine kinase (CK) levels and subacute symmetrical proximal muscular weakness is present in all patients [9]. The typical skin rash as in JDM is less common and due to the slowly progressive course in some patients and the development of muscle atrophy,limb-girdle muscular dystrophy may be presumed [10]. Pathophysiologically, perturbed proteostasis accompanied by an increase of sarcoplasmic chaperones, lysosomal proteins, and aggregation markers was described independently of the antibody status [11,12].

To date, no standardized therapy procedures exist, and some expert recommendations suggest that rituximab should be used in anti-SRP54 and anti-HMGCR Ab positive patients who fail to respond to steroids and intravenous immunoglobulins (IVIG) as second line treatments [13,14]. Patients with anti-SRP54 Ab tend to have a more severe disease course compared to anti-HMGCR Ab positive patients. Younger age at disease onset is associated with more severe symptoms that can be resistant to treatment and therefore poorer prognosis [6,15]. Recent case series in children with anti-SRP54 Ab implicate that an early and intensive combination of immunosuppressive therapy and physiotherapy may lead to early stabilization of the disease and better outcome, although long-term observational studies are still lacking [16]. Similar escalation in therapy was applied in juvenile patients with anti-HMGCR Ab myopathy in cases of severe weakness [2,5], but in some mild-affected cases, IVIG monotherapy led to remission and normalization of CK-levels [10].

Here, we describe the clinical and myopathological findings as well as the therapeutic challenges of two pediatric patients with IMNM on long-term follow up. In both, due to profound muscle weakness and the undulating course of the disease, it was difficult to determine the most suitable moment to adjust, terminate, or escalate the respective therapies. Of note, in the long term, both patients developed muscular atrophy and persisting muscular weakness.

2. Materials and Methods

2.1. Patient Recruitment

We recruited one patient from the Neuromuscular Center, Department of Child Neurology, Children's Hospital, University Hospital Essen and one from the Department for Neurology—Institute of Translational Neurology, University Hospital Münster, Germany. All data concerning Patients 1 and 2 were extracted retrospectively from their medical files.

2.2. Antibody Analyses

Screening for myositis specific antibodies (Abs) was performed with line blot commercial immunoassays (Labor Berlin, Berlin, Labor Euroimmun, Luebeck, Germany) and included the Mi-2alpha und beta, TIF1g, MDA5, NXP2, Ku, PM-Scl 100/75, SRP, Jo-1, PL-7, PL-12, EJ, OJ, SAE, Ro-52. B, U1-RNP, Sm, SS-a/Ro-52, SS-B, Scl70, and CENP-B. Negative controls were used for the applied assay. Anti-HMGCR Ab was detected using a commercial Enzyme Linked Immunosorbent Assay (ELISA, Labor Volkmann, Karlsruhe, Germany).

2.3. Muscle Biopsy Investigations

Biopsies were obtained for diagnostic procedures including histology, enzyme histochemistry, immunofluorescence, and immunohistochemical investigations. Serial cryosections (10 µm) of transversely oriented muscle blocks were stained according to standard procedures with hematoxylin and eosin (H&E), Gömöri trichrome (GT), COX-SDH and SDH and nicotinamide adenine dinucleotide tetrazolium reductase (NADH-TR).

Immunofluorescence studies were performed using antibodies against α-Dystroglycan (α-DG) (Millipore #05-593, clone IIH6C4, 1:10), CD4 (Zytomed, clone SP35, ready-to-use), CD8 (DAKO, clone C8/144B, 1:100), CD68 (DAKO, clone EBM11, 1:100), MHC class I (DAKO, clone W6/32 1:1000), MHC class II (DAKO, clone CR3/43, 1:100), C5b-9 (DAKO/M777, clone aE11, 1:100) (data not shown). Immunofluorescence staining was performed in staining chambers after fixation in acetone for 10 min. The sections were then blocked with the appropriate serum (1:10 in PBS), dependent on the source of the secondary antibody, and incubated with the aforementioned primary antibodies over night at 4 °C or for 1 h at room temperature. After a washing step, the secondary antibody was added for 1 h. After a final washing step, the sections were aqueously mounted and stored at 4 °C.

Immunohistochemistry was conducted using antibodies against αB-crystallin (Abcam, ab13496, 1:2.500, mouse, clone 1B6.1-3G4), HSP70 (Abcam, ab6535, 1:100, mouse, clone BRM-22), LC3 (Nanotools Art, 0260-100, 1:50, mouse, clone LC3-2G6), LAMP2 (Santa Cruz Biotechnology, USA, SC-18822, 1:500, mouse, clone 5H2), and p62 (Abcam, ab91526, 1:100, rabbit, polyclonal). These immunoreactions were performed using the iVIEW-Ventana DAB (diaminobenzidine)-Detection Kit (Ventana, Tucson, AD, USA, 85755 USA). Appropriate biotinylated secondary antibodies were used, and visualization of the reaction product was carried out on a Benchmark XT immunostainer (Ventana) in a standardized manner. Cellular structures were counterstained with hematoxylin.

We used normal muscle tissue as a negative control (or physiological internal control, e.g., staining of major histocompatability class I (MHC class I) positivity of capillaries) for all reactions. Light microscopic investigations were performed using a Zeiss Axioplan epifluorescence microscope equipped with a Zeiss Axio Cam ICc1 and a Zeiss, BZ-X800 microscope (software: BZ-X800 Viewer).

3. Results
3.1. Clinical Presentations
3.1.1. Patient 1

The patient was born after an uneventful pregnancy, delivery and postnatal period were normal. She was age-adequately psychomotorically developed. At 8 years of age, signs of proximal muscular weakness occurred over a period of 8 months: her strength declined rapidly, and she was not able to climb stairs or to lift from the sitting position. Her maximum walking distance was 20 m. She developed dysphagia with swallowing difficulties and weight loss; restrictive pulmonary function with reduced coughing strength and forced vital capacity (FVC: 78%) were present. The childhood myositis assessment scale (CMAS) reflected her muscular weakness, with a score of 4/52 points. Laboratory findings showed raised CK of 10.710 U/L (50–240 U/L), LDH of 2.260 U/L (380–640 U/L), ASL of 336 U/L (<50 U/L), ALT of 310 U/L (10–45 U/L), and aldolase of 127 U/L (y7,6 U/L). CRP was negative. Cardial investigations (echocardiography, electrocardiogram) revealed normal results. In another clinic, due to lack of cutaneous signs for dermatomyositis, muscular dystrophy was first assumed, and investigation of a tailored genetic panel revealed no pathological mutation in the included genes (*ANO5, CAPN3, CAV3, DYSF, FKRP, GAA, MYOT, PYGM, SGCA, SGCB, SGCD, SGCG, TCAP*). No skin lesions were present at onset. Muscle magnetic resonance imaging (MRI) showed a symmetrical, patchy, elevated T2-weighted short tau inversion recovery (STIR) signal in the muscles of the pelvis, both thighs, and lower legs (Figure 1A).

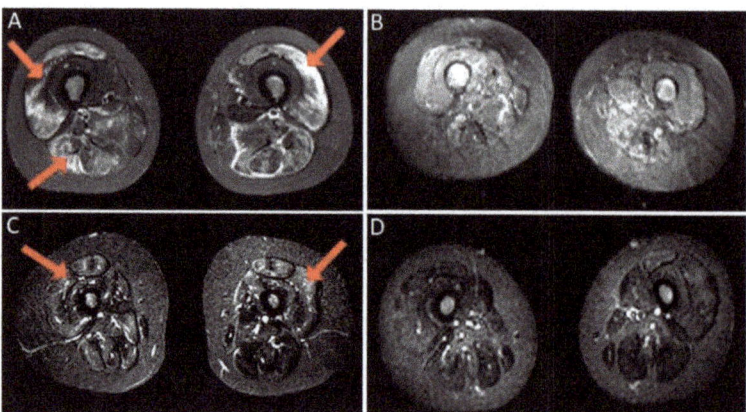

Figure 1. Magnetic resonance imaging (MRI) of both patients using the short tau inversion recovery (STIR) sequence. Patient 1: patchy, symmetrical edema of the thigh muscles at onset (**A**, arrows) and normalization of the STIR signal as well as marked fatty atrophy of the previously affected thigh muscles after one year of therapy (**B**). MRI–STIR sequence of Patient 2: patchy signal elevation predominantly in the quadriceps muscles, left more pronounced than the right, 4 months after starting therapy (**C**, arrows). Reduced signal elevations and atrophy of the quadriceps muscles at 10-year follow up (**D**).

In myositis-panel analyses, positivity for SRP54-Ab was detected and therapy with pulsed methylprednisolone intravenous (IV) in combination with oral prednisolone and methotrexate was started. Under this therapy, her bulbar symptoms improved, but no improvement in her muscular strength was achieved although her CK levels decreased during the period of 3 months (1.639 U/L). Therefore, the therapy was switched to monthly IVIG (2 g/kg). Under this combination, her CK levels normalized, and her CMAS score improved to 36/52 12 months afterwards. She presented almost normal muscular strength in her lower extremities but developed persistent, asymmetrical weakness and atrophy in her upper extremities (Figure 2A–C). Her bulbar symptoms completely reversed, but her axial muscular weakness persisted. Her CK levels were within the normal range 15 months post-therapy start, and MRI follow up showed normalization of the T2 weighted STIR signal but revealed marked fatty atrophy of the previously affected muscles (Figure 1B). After two months, her CK-levels increased again (392 U/L), but her CMAS score remained stable. Due to the further increase in her CK levels and persistent weakness in her upper extremities as well as atrophy, therapy with rituximab was started. After two months, she developed severe weakness, her CK levels increased significantly (4.973 U/L), and her CMAS dropped to 8/52. Additionally, she developed a skin rash (Figure 2D), and oral steroid therapy was re-started. With this combination, she improved again, achieving a CMAS score of 26/52. She received rituximab three times (375 mg/m^2), and within 7 months, a normalization of her CK levels was achieved. Due to a lack of improvement, methotrexate-treatment was stopped, and she remained on therapy with IVIG. Her CK levels rose again, and a fourth dose of rituximab was applied (Figure 3). Her CMAS score remained at 29/52, and her CK levels normalized. At the end of follow up, she was able to walk a distance of over 1000 m, but she had to hold onto a railing when climbing stairs and had positive Gower's phenomena when rising up from the floor, but she was able to stand up from the sitting position unsupported.

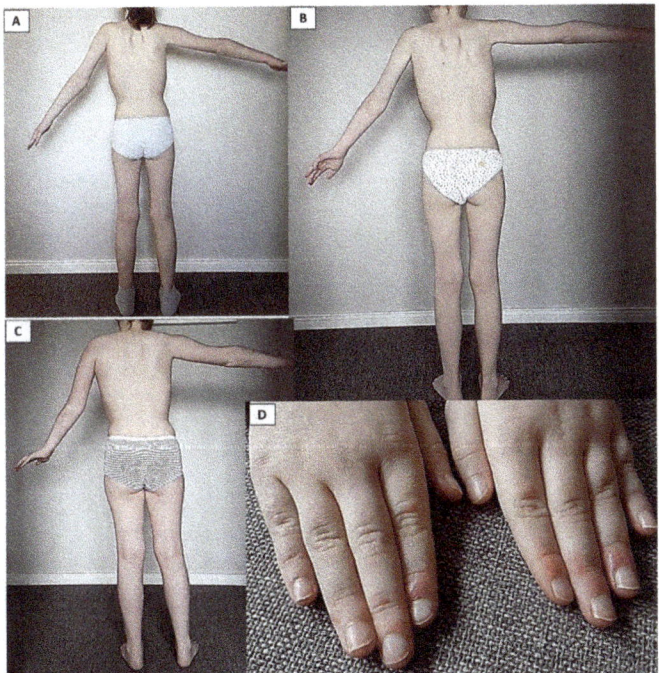

Figure 2. Patient 1 presenting asymmetrical weakness in her upper extremities. The patient presents the highest active elevation of her arms: (**A**): 3 months after methlyprednisolone intravenous therapy in combination with oral steroids and methotrexate; (**B**): 20-month follow up (rituximab, intravenous immunoglobulins, and methotrexate). The strength in her right arm was better compared to her left arm. Asymmetrical weakness persisted at the 2 years and 7 months follow up (**C**), and she developed skin lesions for the first time (periungual exanthema) (**D**).

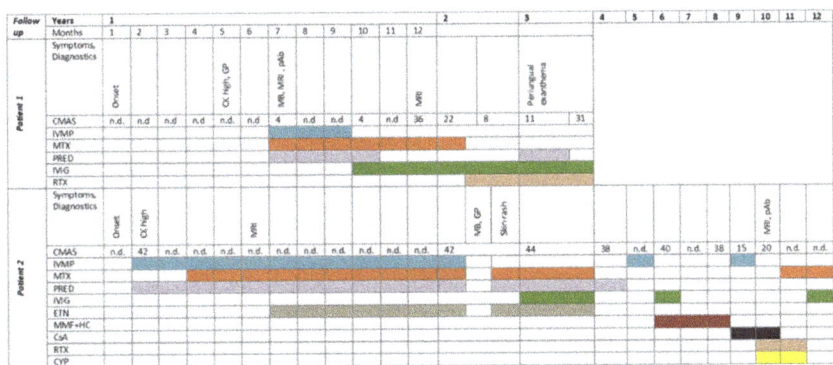

Figure 3. Timelines of both juvenile IMNM patients including onset of symptoms, diagnostics, and applied therapies. Patient 1 was followed for 3 years, and Patient 2 was followed for over 10 years. CMAS = childhood myositis assessment scale, maximal 52 points, CK = creatine kinase, GP = genetic panel, MB = muscular biopsy, MRI = magnetic resonance imaging, CsA = cyclosporine A, CYP = cyclophosphamide, ETN = etanercept, IVMP = intravenous methylprednisolone, MMF + HC = mycophenolate mofetile and hydroxychloroquine, MTX = methotrexate, PRED = prednisolone, RTX = rituximab, Onset = symptom onset, n.d. = not done, pAb = positive antibodies.

3.1.2. Patient 2

The mother´s pregnancy and birth of the female patient were uneventful. She showed age-adequate psychomotor development. At the age of 9 years, signs of proximal muscular weakness occurred, and over the period of 1 month her muscle strength declined rapidly and she presented with increasing difficulties when climbing stairs. Her CMAS score was 42/52 points. She had proximal muscle weakness and had to hold onto railing when climbing stairs. In addition, she suffered from high fever for several days before her first hospital admission. An MRI of the thighs after 4 months of therapy showed patchy signal enhancement predominantly in both quadriceps muscles (left > right, Figure 1C). Laboratory findings showed raised serum CK of 18.000 U/L (50–240 U/L), LDH of 1.862 U/L (380–640 U/L), AST of 532 U/L (<50 U/L), and ALT of 900 U/L (10–45 U/L). CRP was negative. Cardial investigations (echocardiography, electrocardiogram) revealed normal results. Moreover, skin exanthema appeared in the neck region. A biopsy of the skin revealed suspected interstitial granulomatous dermatitis without typical findings for dermatomyositis.

Under the suspicion of a JDM, treatment was initiated with pulsed methylprednisolone IV (20 mg/kg/day on three consecutive days) every 2nd week for 3 months and once/month afterwards. Additionally, she received 5 mg oral prednisolone in combination with methotrexate (15 mg/m^2 weekly) (Figure 3). After six months, etanercept (25 mg/day) was added due to persistent clinical symptoms with proximal limb weakness, highly elevated serum CK (3.932 U/L), and radiological signs of inflammation in both quadriceps muscles. Her muscular strength improved over the 12-month period, but she developed reduced muscular endurance (CMAS 44/52). Immunosuppressive therapy was stopped due to negative screening for myositis-specific Abs (HMGCR Ab was not included in the panel), and muscular dystrophy was assumed. A muscle biopsy showed myopathic features, and staining of α-dystrogycan protein fragments showed a mosaic pattern of α-dystrogycan-positive and α-dystrogylcan-negative fibres with scattered lympho-monocytic infiltrates (Figure 4D). Commercial genetic panel testing for common dystroglycanopathy genes was negative (*FKRP, FKTN, POMT1, ISDP, DYSF*).

After another two months, she developed a typical skin rash (on her finger extensor regions and on her trunk), and immunosuppression was restarted (prednisolone, methotrexate and etanercept) (Figure 3). Unfortunately, the patient showed signs of steroid induced osteonecrosis on both femurs, so therapy with pulsed IV methylprednisolone was discontinued, and therapy with IVIG was given over period of 9 months (2 g/kg every month). With this treatment regime, muscle strength improved significantly in both limbs. However, as relevant deficits persisted (CMAS 40/52), treatment with methotrexate and etanercept was discontinued, and therapy with mycophenolate mofetil (2 × 500 mg/day) was initiated in combination with hydroxychloroquine, followed by another treatment switch after one year (cyclosporine A). Her CK levels remained high (2.773 U/L). After a clinically stable period of 2 years, a rapid clinical deterioration (CMAS 15/52) was observed. Therefore, she received additional steroid pulse therapy every month for half a year without relevant clinical improvement. Further diagnostics were initiated with screening for further myositis-specific Abs, including HMGCR-Ab for the first time. The latter was repeatedly highly elevated >200 U/mL (<20 U/mL). MRI control (10 years after the first symptoms) showed atrophy in both quadriceps muscles with only sparse inflammation (Figure 1D). HMGCR-Ab positive IMNM was diagnosed, and the patient received rituximab as monotherapy, resulting in clinical stabilization after three cycles (CMAS 19/52). Unfortunately, 3 months after the last cycle, a rapid decrease of muscle strength in both legs was documented, resulting in a further treatment switch to IV cyclophosphamide (350–500 mg/m^2) every month. Although disease stability was achieved, therapy with cyclophosphamide was stopped after 19 cycles due to persistent lymphopenia. Again, a treatment regime with methotrexate and IVIG was initiated after the lymphocyte normalization (Figure 3).

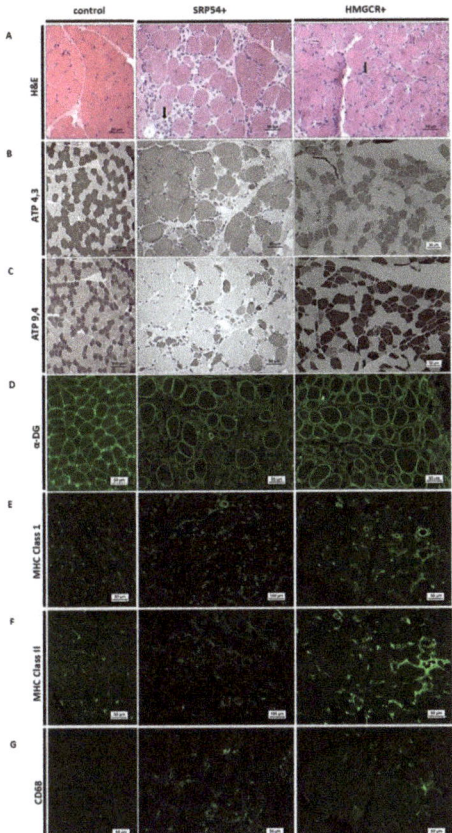

Figure 4. Muscle biopsy findings in pediatric IMNM patients; the middle column seropositive patient for SRP54, and the right column is seropositive patient for HMGCR. Patient 1 (SRP54+): perimysial proliferation of connective tissue (**A**, white arrow) is detectable but no lymphohistiocytic cell infiltrates are observed. Moreover, marked fibre size variability with numerous atrophic fibres are present (**A**, black arrow). Increased type 1 fibres and predominantly atrophic type-2 fibres (**B**,**C**) are identified by ATPase staining. Immunofluorescence studies revealed α-dystroglycan-positive and α-dystroglycan-negative necrotic fibres (**D**). Moreover, major histocompatibility class I (MHC class I) immunoreactivity is increased in degenerating fibers in addition to a non-specific reactivity at the sarcolemma and within the sarcoplasm of many fibres (**E**). Along this line, MHC II is markedly increased at the vessels, subsarcolemmally, and in necrotic fibres (**F**). Foci of regeneration are associated with small basophilic fibres and with large nuclei clusters of regenerating fibres that are also admixed with many macrophages (CD68-positive) (**G**). Patient 2 (HMGCR+): H&E staining revealed marked fibre size variability and hypertrophy, grouped atrophic fibers (black arrow), diffuse cell necrosis, and phagocytosis as well as basophilic regenerating fibres often clustering in groups (**A**). Immunofluorescence studies of the α-dystroglycan protein fragments showed a mosaic pattern of α-dystroglycan-positive and α-dystroglycan-negative fibres (**D**). MHC class I and II upregulation is present perivascular and only rarely present subsarcolemmally (**E**,**F**). Increased CD68 expression is detectable in the perivascular region and in necrotic fibres (**G**).

3.2. Muscle Biopsy Findings

To assess the pathology of skeletal muscle in pediatric IMNM patients, we examined general histological alterations in the biopsies of two patients. Small, mostly rounded fibres were identified accompanied by increased variation in fibre size and increased fibrosis in the endomysium as well as enlargement of the perimysium (on H&E, Figure 4A). Foci of regeneration with small basophilic fibres with large nuclei clusters of regenerating fibres were admixed with many macrophages and some lymphocytes in Patient 1 (Figure 4A, SRP+). Additionally, we identified that the staining of α-dystroglycan protein fragments showed a mosaic pattern of α-dystroglycan-positive and α-dystroglycan-negative fibres in Patient 2 (Figure 4D, HMGC+). Major histocompatibility class I (MHC class I) immunoreactivity was increased in the degenerating fibres and nonspecifically on the sarcolemma and the sarcoplasm of many fibres (Figure 4E). In addition, MHC II immunoreactivity was increased at the vessels, subsarcolemally, and in necrotic fibres (Figure 4F). Regeneration foci with small basophilic fibres with large nuclei clusters of regenerating fibres were admixed with many macrophages (Figure 4A,G).

To investigate if juvenile IMNM patients share the pathophysiological cascades that are known to take place in adult cases, we next focused on proteostasis by immunological examination of biochemical markers including chaperones, protein clearance proteins, and a protein aggregation marker known to be increased in adult IMNM patients [11]. We therefore chose some markers that are crucially involved in the chaperone-assisted selective autophagy (CASA) pathway. Staining of HSP70 and αB-crystallin demonstrated clear upregulation in both patients, whereby the intensity of HSP70 staining in the HMGCR patient was less strong (Figure 5A,B). Lysosomal staining with LAMP2 additionally revealed diffuse sarcoplasmic stains with the same intensity in both patients, showing high autophagy activity. No clustering in the perifascicular regions or specific parts of the fascicle could be seen (Figure 5C).

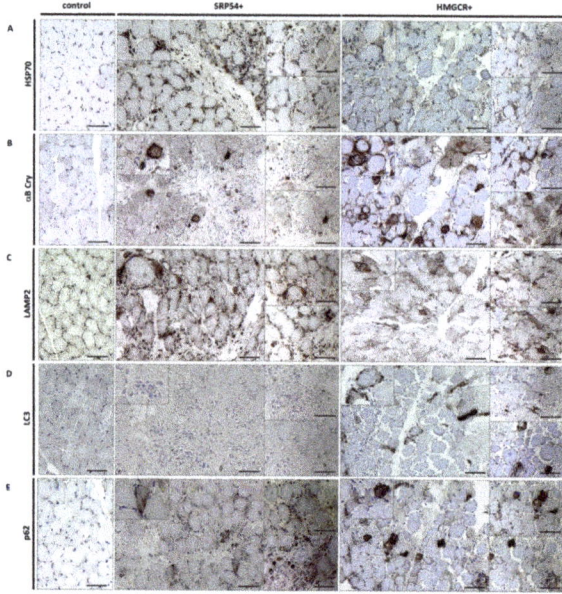

Figure 5. Histological findings in both juvenile IMNM patients with focus on the protein clearance machinery. Histological staining of markers involved in proteostasis showed upregulation of all investigated proteins in both juvenile IMNM patients, with subtle differences in staining intensity. (**A**): HSP70 and (**B**): αB-crystallin show clear upregulation in both patients as well as (**C**): LAMP2, which is stained diffusely on the sarcoplasm. (**D**): LC3 shows a fine granular pattern and is stronger in the HMGCR+ patient, while (**E**): p62 is intense in both patients. A typical pattern in IMNM patients is seen. Necrotic muscle fibres stain is unspecific for all markers. Scale bar = 100 μm.

As previously shown in adult patients [12], the staining pattern of LC3+ and p62+ muscle fibres show a fine granular pattern throughout the entire sarcoplasm, which is common for IMNM patients and can also be seen in both juvenile patients (Figure 5D,E). Especially in the SRP54+ patient, numerous fibres are intensely immunoreactive for p62.

4. Discussion

IMNM in children is a rare but is relevant differential diagnosis to juvenile dermatomyositis and presents a diagnostic challenge due to mostly lacking typical cutaneous manifestations and only partial response to first line immunosuppressive therapy with steroids and methotrexate. The increased level of CK values or typical findings indicative for myositis on the MRI level do not always occur simultaneously in combination with clinical aggravation in our patients; this, in turn, makes the decision when to change or escalate therapy challenging.

4.1. Comparison to Previously Reported Juvenile and Adult IMNM Cases

In adult patients with anti-SRP54 and anti-HMGCR positive Abs, acute-to-subacute, symmetrical progressive proximal weakness is present in both subgroups and muscular weakness affects the legs more than the arms [6]. However, anti-SRP54 Ab positive patients have more neck weakness and dysphagia compared to HMGCR-Ab patients. Consistent with this, Patient 1 in our study presented with bulbar symptoms at disease onset. Muscular atrophy was significantly more present in SRP54-seropositive cases compared to HMGCR-positive patients, although it seems that a longer active disease period also leads to muscular atrophy in the latter group [6,10]. Of note, younger adult patients had a more severe disease course accompanied by a worse prognosis compared to older patients in long-term follow-up studies [6,15]. A similar presentation as in adults, but with additional distal weakness, was also reported in a small population of pediatric patients with SRP54- and HMGCR-Ab positive serostatus. Interestingly, muscular atrophy in combination with mild to moderate muscular weakness despite intensive therapy was present in 86–100%, which is higher compared to other myositis-specific Abs [5]. This clinical aspect could also be observed in our patients, who both presented muscular atrophy at the last follow up, and, in the case of the anti-SRP54 positive patient, already early in the course of the disease. The anti-SRP54 positive patient also had asymmetrical muscle weakness, which so far has not been reported as a specific symptom, and, in case of our patient, asymmetric weakness remained despite intensive therapy during long-term follow up (Figure 2A–C).

4.2. Microscopic Findings

In both patients, the presence of a genetically based muscular dystrophy was suspected at the beginning or during the course of the disease. This suspicion arose due to the unsatisfactory response to immunosuppressive therapy and a lack of specific Abs in the first testing period (Patient 2) and the clinical presentation with absent dermatomyositis-like cutaneous symptoms (both patients) at onset as well as based on the asymmetric muscle weakness (Patient 1). In the group with mostly adult IMNM-patients, necrosis and regeneration of muscle fibres and endomysial fibrosis with no or little endomysial lymphocyte infiltration was present [6,10]. This pathomorphological observation was also present in 2/3 juvenile SRP54-Ab positive patients, comparable with the findings in Patient 1 in our study (Figure 4A). In one patient, inflammatory infiltrates were additionally present, implicating an autoimmune disorder [16]. Moreover, in Patient 2, muscular dystrophy was assumed based on the histologic findings and α-dystrogycan-negative fibres. The misdirection toward a limb-girdle muscular dystrophy (LGMD) has been described previously [10]. In a small group of six HMGCR-Ab positive patients with a longer period of disease duration (3.5 to 23 years), muscle histology showed chronic myopathic features, such as myofibre atrophy, fibre size variability, splitting myofibres, and increased endomysial fibrosis. However, no signs of primary inflammation were present [10]. Similar as in our patient, all patients underwent prior to diagnosis genetic testing for common LGMDs, and in two patients, facioscapulohumeral dystrophy was assumed due to asymmetrical weakness [10].

The histological and immunohistochemistry findings in Patient 1 are comparable to those seen in adults with IMNM. As in adults, the focus is not on the inflammatory process with endomysial lymphocytic inflammation surrounding non-necrotic myofibre, as is the case in JDM, but on fibrous necrosis and macrophage activation with sparse inflammatory infiltrates [6,8,13]. In the Patient 2, muscle biopsy presented more of a myopathic picture, which is not primarily related to IMNM, but has rarely been described in juvenile and adult patients with positive for HMGCR [10,17,18].

Immunostaining studies focusing on proteins known to modulate protein clearance and to be upregulated in adult IMNM patients [11] revealed an increase of sarcoplasmic chaperones (HSP70 and αB-crystallin), modulators of autophagy (LAMP2 and LC3), and a protein aggregation marker (p62), thus also indicating perturbed proteostasis in the disease cause of juvenile patients and along this line confirm the pathophysiological findings described by Preuße and co-workers [11,12]. Given that the modulation of proteostasis is a well-known therapeutic target in a variety of neuromuscular disorders (e.g., [19,20]), by applying chemical chaperones and/or autophagy inducers, our finding might open new avenues for additional therapeutic concepts. In this context it is important to note that several of these drugs are already FDA approved.

4.3. Therapeutic Regimen/Outcome

Taken together, data reported in the literature and our own clinical observations indicate that anti-HMGCR Ab patients tend to have a less progressive disease course and better response to therapy: anti-HMGCR patients responded better to steroid therapy compared to anti-SRP54-seropositive patients, with a higher frequency of steroid monotherapy in the anti-HMGCR group [6]. In both groups, therapy with IVIG is recommended in case of a failed response to steroids or a severe disease course [13]. An early intensive therapy with IVIG, methotrexate, and rituximab and/or cyclophosphamide prevented further progression and even improved clinical symptoms in a small pediatric case series of three patients with anti-SRP54 Ab and a follow-up period of 20–50 weeks [16]. Both of our patients only showed partial and unsatisfactory response to pulse methylprednisolone therapy in combination with methotrexate or etanercept. Under IVIG-treatment, both achieved a longer period of stability (Patient 1 one year, Patient 2 two years in combination with additional immunosuppression), but this was not effective in the long term. Patient 1 showed a renewed increase in CK levels without simultaneous worsening of the CMAS score; this raises the question of reacting to rising CK values in these patients by intensifying the therapy before the clinical symptoms worsen. We also assume that a longer follow-up period is needed for a final assessment of the influence of the therapy due to the undulating course of the disease.

In patients with HMGCR Abs, however, there seems to be a small group that shows little clinical activity over a longer period of time; here, the extent of muscle atrophy seems to be an important parameter to predict the response to therapy [10]. Remarkably, this could be observed also in our patient with a steady state under IVIG therapy for two years, but the further progression of muscular weakness with the development of atrophy and only a partial response to further escalation with rituximab and cyclophosphamide.

Interestingly, in Patient 2, muscular symptoms worsened after respiratory infection with fever, implicating some role of additional inflammation as a possible disease activating factor. In reported SRP54-positive cases, infection or coryzal illness preceded in more than half of the cases at the onset of muscular weakness [16,21–23].

5. Conclusions

In children with a new onset of symmetrical or asymmetrical muscle weakness without cutaneous features associated with dermatomyositis, remarkably high CK-levels, and previously inconspicuous psychomotor development, the presence of inflammatory myopathy should be considered since the appropriate therapeutic options exist in contrast to genetically determined muscular dystrophies. Anti-HMGCR Ab is not always included in the commercial myositis panel, and this possibility must be considered in combination with specific clinical, MRI, and muscle biopsy findings. We believe that in the case of IMNM, clinical presentation in combination with the detection of specific antibodies, MRI changes and muscle biopsy will allow a correct and rapid diagnosis that allows an early start of therapy. In this population, an early and intensive therapy may be crucial for outcome in long-term. Patients should be followed for a long period of time due to the undulating course of the disease, and the worsening of muscular strength and persistently high CK-levels should implicate early escalation or re-start of the immunosuppression. Consistent with adult IMNM, juvenile IMNM-patients also present with perturbed proteostasis, a biochemical observation that might open new avenues for the application of novel therapeutic concepts in the future.

Author Contributions: Conceptualization, A.D.M.; clinical investigation and data curation, A.D.M., M.P., N.V., B.S. and H.K.; myopathological investigations, S.H. and U.S.-S.; C.P. provided the protein clearance data; writing—original draft preparation, A.D.M., M.P. and A.R.; writing—review and editing, A.D.M., M.P., T.R., A.v.B., N.V., B.S., S.H., H.K., H.W., C.P., A.R., U.S.-S. All authors have read and agreed to the published version of the manuscript.

Funding: Parts of this study were financed in the framework of the NME-GPS project by the European Regional Development Fund (ERDF).

Institutional Review Board Statement: The study was conducted according to the guidelines of the Declaration of Helsinki and approved by local Ethics Committee (19-9011-BO). The approval date was 30 April 2020.

Informed Consent Statement: For all diagnostic steps in both patients and in the pictures of the Patient 1, written informed consent has been obtained from the parents of both patients to publish this paper.

Data Availability Statement: The data that support the findings of this study are available from the corresponding author upon reasonable request.

Acknowledgments: The authors thank the patients and their families for their cooperation and for their permission to publish the data and the photographs.

Conflicts of Interest: The authors declare no conflict of interest.

References

1. Yasin, S.A.; Schutz, P.W.; Deakin, C.T.; Sag, E.; Varsani, H.; Simou, S.; Marshall, L.R.; Tansley, S.L.; McHugh, N.J.; Holton, J.L.; et al. Histological heterogeneity in a large clinical cohort of juvenile idiopathic inflammatory myopathy: Analysis by myositis autoantibody and pathological features. *Neuropathol. Appl. Neurobiol.* **2019**, *45*, 495–512. [CrossRef]
2. Tansley, S.L.; Betteridge, Z.E.; Simou, S.; Jacques, T.S.; Pilkington, C.; Wood, M.; Warrier, K.; Wedderburn, L.R.; Mchugh, N.J. Anti-HMGCR Autoantibodies in Juvenile Idiopathic Inflammatory Myopathies Identify a Rare but Clinically Important Subset of Patients. *J. Rheumatol.* **2017**, *44*, 488–492. [CrossRef]
3. Mendez, E.P.; Lipton, R.; Ramsey-Goldman, R.; Roettcher, P.; Bowyer, S.; Dyer, A.; Pachman, L.M. US incidence of juvenile dermatomyositis, 1995-1998: Results from the National Institute of Arthritis and Musculoskeletal and Skin Diseases Registry. *Arthritis Care Res.* **2003**, *49*, 300–305. [CrossRef]
4. Rider, L.G.; Shah, M.; Mamyrova, G.; Huber, A.M.; Rice, M.M.; Targoff, I.N.; Miller, F.W. The Myositis Autoantibody Phenotypes of the Juvenile Idiopathic Inflammatory Myopathies. *Medicine* **2013**, *92*, 223–243. [CrossRef] [PubMed]
5. Kishi, T.; Rider, L.G.; Pak, K.; Barillas-Arias, L.; Henrickson, M.; Mccarthy, P.L.; Shaham, B.; Weiss, P.F.; Horkayne-Szakaly, I.; Targoff, I.N.; et al. Anti-3-Hydroxy-3-Methylglutaryl-Coenzyme A Reductase Autoantibodies are Associated with DRB1*07:01 and Severe Myositis in Pediatric Myositis Patients HHS Public Access. *Arthritis Care Res* **2017**, *69*, 1088–1094. [CrossRef] [PubMed]
6. Watanabe, Y.; Uruha, A.; Suzuki, S.; Nakahara, J.; Hamanaka, K.; Takayama, K.; Suzuki, N.; Nishino, I. Clinical features and prognosis in anti-SRP and anti-HMGCR necrotising myopathy. *J. Neurol. Neurosurg. Psychiatry* **2016**, *87*, 1038–1044. [CrossRef]
7. Ladislau, L.; Arouche-Delaperche, L.; Allenbach, Y.; Benveniste, O. Potential Pathogenic Role of Anti-Signal Recognition Protein and Anti-3-hydroxy-3-methylglutaryl-CoA Reductase Antibodies in Immune-Mediated Necrotizing Myopathies. *Curr. Rheumatol. Rep.* **2018**, *20*, 1–7. [CrossRef] [PubMed]
8. Stenzel, W.; Goebel, H.H.; Aronica, E. Review: Immune-mediated necrotizing myopathies—A heterogeneous group of diseases with specific myopathological features. *Neuropathol. Appl. Neurobiol.* **2012**, *38*, 632–646. [CrossRef] [PubMed]

9. Pinal-Fernandez, I.; Casal-Dominguez, M.; Mammen, A.L. Immune-Mediated Necrotizing Myopathy. *Curr. Rheumatol. Rep.* **2018**, *20*, 1–10. [CrossRef]
10. Mohassel, P.; Landon-Cardinal, O.; Reghan Foley, A.; Donkervoort, S.; Pak, K.S.; Wahl, C.; Shebert, R.T.; Harper, A.; Fequiere, P.; Meriggioli, M.; et al. Anti-HMGCR myopathy may resemble limb-girdle muscular dystrophy. *Intern. Med. Clin. Immunol.* **2019**, *6*, e523. [CrossRef]
11. Preuße, C.; Goebel, H.H.; Held, J.; Wengert, O.; Scheibe, F.; Irlbacher, K.; Koch, A.; Heppner, F.L.; Stenzel, W. Immune-mediated necrotizing myopathy is characterized by a specific Th1-M1 polarized immune profile. *Am. J. Pathol.* **2012**, *181*, 2161–2171. [CrossRef]
12. Fischer, N.; Preuße, C.; Radke, J.; Pehl, D.; Allenbach, Y.; Schneider, U.; Feist, E.; von Casteleyn, V.; Hahn, K.; Ruck, T.; et al. Sequestosome-1 (p62) expression reveals chaperone-assisted selective autophagy in immune-mediated necrotizing myopathies. *Brain Pathol.* **2020**, *30*, 261–271. [CrossRef] [PubMed]
13. Allenbach, Y.; Mammen, A.L.; Benveniste, O.; Stenzel, W.; Allenbach, Y.; Amato, A.; Aussey, A.; Benveniste, O.; De Bleecker, J.; de Groot, I.; et al. 224th ENMC International Workshop: Clinico-sero-pathological classification of immune-mediated necrotizing myopathies. In Proceedings of the Neuromuscular Disorders, Zandvoort, The Netherlands, 14–16 October 2016; Volume 28, pp. 87–99.
14. Schmidt, J. Current Classification and Management of Inflammatory Myopathies. *J. Neuromuscul. Dis.* **2018**, *5*, 109–129. [CrossRef]
15. Tiniakou, E.; Pinal-Fernandez, I.; Lloyd, T.E.; Albayda, J.; Paik, J.; Werner, J.L.; Parks, C.A.; Casciola-Rosen, L.; Christopher-Stine, L.; Mammen, A.L. More severe disease and slower recovery in younger patients with anti-3-hydroxy-3-methylglutarylcoenzyme A reductase-associated autoimmune myopathy. *Rheumatology* **2017**, *56*, 787–794. [PubMed]
16. Binns, E.L.; Moraitis, E.; Maillard, S.; Tansley, S.; McHugh, N.; Jacques, T.S.; Wedderburn, L.R.; Pilkington, C.; Yasin, S.A.; Nistala, K.; et al. Effective induction therapy for anti-SRP associated myositis in childhood: A small case series and review of the literature. *Pediatr. Rheumatol.* **2017**, *15*, 77. [CrossRef]
17. Liang, W.C.; Uruha, A.; Suzuki, S.; Murakami, N.; Takeshita, E.; Chen, W.Z.; Jong, Y.J.; Endo, Y.; Komaki, H.; Fujii, T.; et al. Pediatric necrotizing myopathy associated with anti-3-hydroxy-3-methylglutaryl-coenzyme A reductase antibodies. *Rheumatology* **2017**, *56*, 287–293. [CrossRef]
18. Mohassel, P.; Mammen, A.L. Anti-HMGCR Myopathy. *J. Neuromuscul. Dis.* **2018**, *5*, 11–20. [CrossRef]
19. Ahmed, M.; MacHado, P.M.; Miller, A.; Spicer, C.; Herbelin, L.; He, J.; Noel, J.; Wang, Y.; McVey, A.L.; Pasnoor, M.; et al. Targeting protein homeostasis in sporadic inclusion body myositis. *Sci. Transl. Med.* **2016**, *8*, 331ra41. [CrossRef]
20. Franekova, V.; Storjord, H.I.; Leivseth, G.; Nilssen, Ø. Protein homeostasis in LGMDR9 (LGMD2I)—The role of ubiquitin–proteasome and autophagy–lysosomal system. *Neuropathol. Appl. Neurobiol.* **2021**, *47*, 519–531. [CrossRef] [PubMed]
21. Momomura, M.; Miyamae, T.; Nozawa, T.; Kikuchi, M.; Kizawa, T.; Imagawa, T.; Drouot, L.; Jouen, F.; Boyer, O.; Yokota, S. Serum levels of anti-SRP54 antibodies reflect disease activity of necrotizing myopathy in a child treated effectively with combinatorial methylprednisolone pulses and plasma exchanges followed by intravenous cyclophosphamide. *Mod. Rheumatol.* **2014**, *24*, 529–531. [CrossRef] [PubMed]
22. Kawabata, T.; Komaki, H.; Saito, T.; Saito, Y.; Nakagawa, E.; Sugai, K.; Sasaki, M.; Hayashi, Y.K.; Nishino, I.; Momomura, M.; et al. A pediatric patient with myopathy associated with antibodies to a signal recognition particle. *Brain Dev.* **2012**, *34*, 877–880. [CrossRef] [PubMed]
23. Rouster-Stevens, K.A.; Pachman, L.M. Autoantibody to signal recognition particle in African American girls with juvenile polymyositis. *J. Rheumatol.* **2008**, *35*, 927–929. [PubMed]

Case Report

Improvement in Fine Manual Dexterity in Children with Spinal Muscular Atrophy Type 2 after Nusinersen Injection: A Case Series

Minsu Gu and Hyun-Ho Kong *

Department of Rehabilitation Medicine, Chungbuk National University Hospital, Cheongju 28644, Korea; msgrehab@gmail.com
* Correspondence: jimlight@hanmail.net

Abstract: Although nusinersen has been demonstrated to improve motor function in patients with spinal muscular atrophy (SMA), no studies have investigated its effect on fine manual dexterity. The present study aimed to investigate the ability of nusinersen to improve fine manual dexterity in patients with SMA type 2. A total of five patients with SMA type 2 were included. The Hammersmith Functional Motor Scale (expanded version) (HFMSE) and Purdue Pegboard (PP) tests were used to evaluate gross motor function and fine manual dexterity, respectively, until 18 months after nusinersen administration. HFMSE scores improved by 3–10 points (+13–53%) in all patients following nusinersen administration. PP scores also improved in all patients, from 4 to 9 points (+80–225%) in the preferred hand and from 3 to 7 points (+60–500%) in the non-preferred hand. These results suggest that nusinersen treatment improved both gross motor function and fine manual dexterity in children with SMA type 2. Addition of the PP test may aid in evaluating the fine manual dexterity essential for activities of daily living in these patients.

Keywords: spinal muscular atrophy (SMA); nusinersen; fine manual dexterity

1. Introduction

Spinal muscular atrophy (SMA) is an autosomal recessive disorder that affects the motor neurons in the anterior horn of the spinal cord, resulting in muscle atrophy and loss of muscle strength [1]. SMA is caused by insufficient production of SMN protein due to deletion or mutation of the survival motor neuron 1 (SMN 1) gene [2,3].

Recently, nusinersen targeting the SMN gene has been used as a treatment for SMA. Previous research has consistently demonstrated that nusinersen treatment improves both gross motor function as measured using the Hammersmith Functional Motor Scale (expanded version) (HFMSE) and upper extremity motor function as measured using the Revised Upper Limb Module (RULM) in patients with later-onset SMA [4].

Although the RULM also includes some items related to hand dexterity, such as picking up coins and tearing a piece of paper, it is difficult to assess quantitative changes in dexterity because the tool utilizes a three-point scale (0, 1, 2). Previous studies only addressed changes in the total RULM score following administration of nusinersen, without performing subgroup analysis for specific items [4,5]. Therefore, while such studies were able to confirm improvements in general upper limb motor function following nusinersen administration, they were unable to confirm whether patients exhibited improvements in fine manual dexterity. The present study is the first to investigate and demonstrate the effect of nusinersen on fine manual dexterity in patients with SMA type 2.

2. Materials and Methods

2.1. Patients

A total of five patients with 5q SMA, confirmed based on SMN1 genetic documentation, were included in this study. All patients had a clinical classification of SMA type 2 and received neither permanent ventilator support nor enteral feeding. Between May 2019 and December 2019, the patients were referred to the Department of Rehabilitation Medicine to evaluate functional changes before and after nusinersen administration.

Nusinersen was administered intrathecally at a dose of 12 mg on days 0 (1st), 14 (2nd), 28 (3rd), and 63 (4th) according to the protocol, following which, it was administered once every 4 months for maintenance. Functional evaluations were performed before starting nusinersen treatment, between the 3rd and 4th doses, and before administration during the maintenance period. Patients underwent follow-up for a total of 18 months.

This study was approved by the Institutional Review Board of Chungbuk National University (CBNUH 2021-08-011), who waived the requirement for informed consent due to the retrospective nature of the study.

2.2. Functional Assessments

The 33-item HFMSE was developed to evaluate gross motor function related to daily living in patients with SMA type 2 or 3. Each item is scored from 0 (no response) to 2 (full response), with total scores ranging from 0 to 66 [6,7].

The Purdue Pegboard (PP) test is a standardized assessment of fine manual dexterity that is mainly used to evaluate functional abnormalities in patients with neurological impairment or developmental delay. There are normative data for most age groups, as well as reference data for preschool children over the age of 2 years, 6 months [8].

The PP test was used to evaluate fine manual dexterity in each hand. The PP test assesses the patient's ability to pick up pegs one at a time from a cup on top of the pegboard and insert them into the holes as quickly as possible. The test was first performed using the preferred hand followed by the non-preferred hand, and the number of pegs inserted within 30 s was measured [8].

The assessments were performed by one trained clinical evaluator, and training was conducted to establish reliability before data collection began.

3. Results

3.1. Baseline Characteristics

Baseline characteristics for the five patients included in the study are summarized in Table 1. All five patients were female and had SMA type 2. Genetic sequencing analysis indicated that the SMN2 gene copy number was 3 in all 5 patients. The age at the onset of SMA symptoms ranged from 12 to 14 months, while the age at SMA diagnosis ranged from 2 to 24 months. The age at initiation of nusinersen treatment ranged from 12 to 14 months (Table 1).

Table 1. Baseline characteristics of the study patients.

Patient Number	Sex	SMA Type	SMN2 Copy Number	Age at Symptom Onset (Month)	Age at Diagnosis (Month)	Age at First Dose (Month)
1	Female	2	3	12	2	58
2	Female	2	3	13	24	82
3	Female	2	3	14	23	40
4	Female	2	3	12	21	38
5	Female	2	3	13	21	65

SMA—spinal muscular atrophy; SMN—survival motor neuron.

3.2. Efficacy Results

3.2.1. Hammersmith Functional Motor Scale (Expanded Version)

Baseline HFMSE scores before nusinersen administration ranged from 10 to 40 points. At 18 months after nusinersen administration, HFMSE scores had improved in all patients, ranging from a minimum of +3 points to a maximum of +10 points (+13–53%). Although there were variations among patients, gross motor functions related to trunk control such as lying, rolling, sitting, crawling, and kneeling [9] tended to improve (Table 2 and Figure 1).

Table 2. Change in HFMSE scores from baseline after nusinersen injection.

Patient Number	Baseline HFMSE Score	Δ Lying and Rolling	Δ Sitting	Δ Crawling and Kneeling	Δ Standing	Δ Walking, Running, and Jumping	HFMSE Score after 7th Dose	Δ HFMSE Score (Δ%)
1	10	+2	+3	0	0	0	15	+5 (+50%)
2	19	+5	+1	+4	0	0	29	+10 (+53%)
3	40	+3	0	+1	+1	+1	46	+6 (+15%)
4	13	0	+3	0	0	0	16	+3 (+23%)
5	30	+3	0	+1	0	0	34	+4 (+13%)

HFMSE—Hammersmith Functional Motor Scale (expanded version); Δ—amount of change.

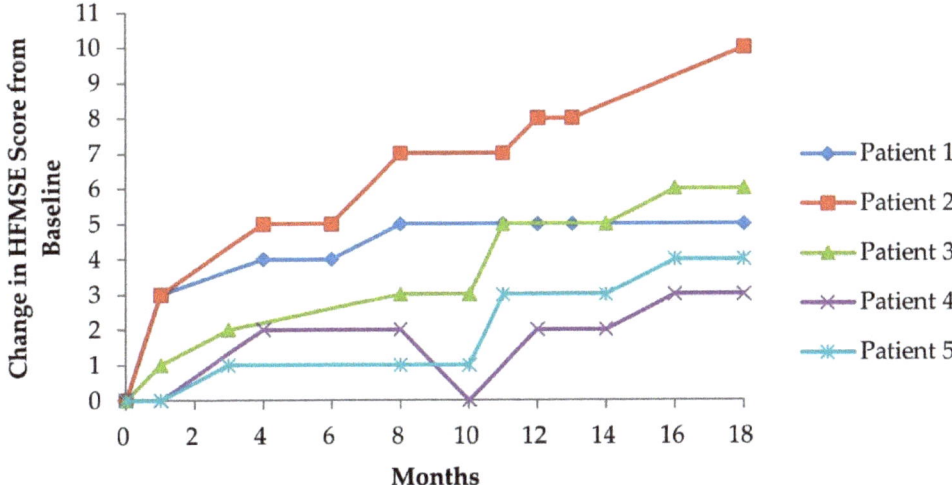

Figure 1. Change in HFMSE score from baseline to 18 months after nusinersen injection. HFMSE—Hammersmith Functional Motor Scale (expanded version).

3.2.2. Purdue Pegboard Test

In the preferred hand, PP scores before and 18 months after the initiation of nusinersen administration ranged from 2 to 7 and from 6 to 14, respectively. The PP score of the preferred hand improved in all patients, ranging from +4 to +9 (+80–225%) when compared with the baseline score (Table 3 and Figure 2a).

In the non-preferred hand, PP scores before and 18 months after the initiation of nusinersen administration ranged from 1 to 6 and from 6 to 13, respectively. The PP score of the non-preferred hand also improved in all patients, ranging from +3 to +7 (+60–500%) when compared with the baseline score (Table 3 and Figure 2b).

Shown in Figure 3, most subjects—except for patient 3—had lower PP scores than normative data of the same age and sex before nusinersen administration; however, the PP scores in both hands of patients 2, 3, and 5 after nusinersen administration (at 18 months) improved to the normal range.

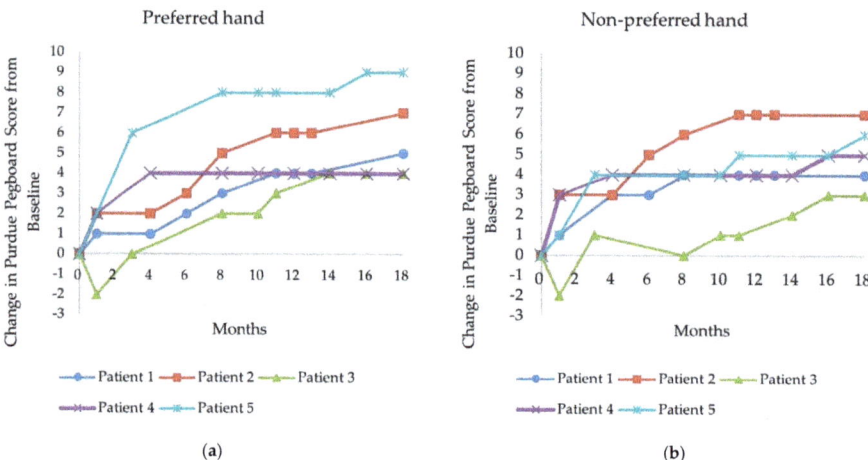

Figure 2. Change in Purdue Pegboard score from baseline to 18 months. (**a**) Preferred hand; (**b**) non-preferred hand.

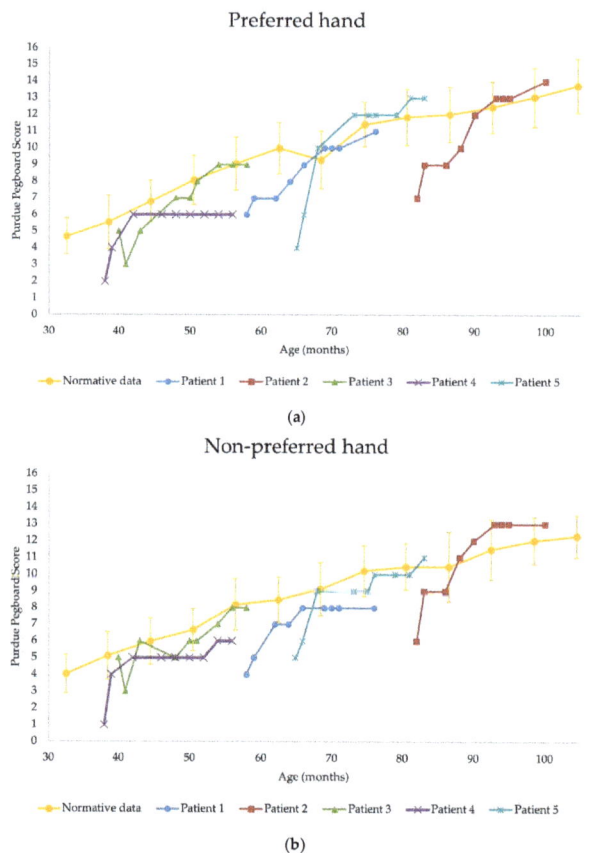

Figure 3. Comparison of Purdue Pegboard score changes in patients versus normative data. (**a**) Preferred hand; (**b**) non-preferred hand.

Table 3. Change in Purdue Pegboard scores from baseline.

Patient Number	Δ HFMSE Score (Δ%)	Preferred Hand PP Score		Non-Preferred Hand PP Score	
		Baseline	After 7th Dose	Baseline	After 7th Dose
1	+5 (+50%)	6	11	4	8
Δ PP score (Δ%)		+5 (+83%)		+4 (+100%)	
2	+10 (+53%)	7	14	6	13
Δ PP score (Δ%)		+7 (+100%)		+7 (+117%)	
3	+6 (+15%)	5	9	5	8
Δ PP score (Δ%)		+4 (+80%)		+3 (+60%)	
4	+3 (+23%)	2	6	1	6
Δ PP score (Δ%)		+4 (+200%)		+5 (+500%)	
5	+4 (+13%)	4	13	5	11
Δ PP score (Δ%)		+9 (+225%)		+6 (+120%)	

HFMSE—Hammersmith Functional Motor Scale (expanded version); PP—Purdue Pegboard; Δ—amount of change.

4. Discussion

In this study, we investigated the effects of nusinersen in five patients with SMA type 2. Gross motor function as measured using the HFMSE improved in all patients after 18 months of treatment, and the functional improvements were mainly related to trunk control. Moreover, fine manual dexterity, as evaluated using the PP test, significantly improved in all patients following nusinersen treatment, and there was no difference between the preferred and non-preferred hands.

In the present study, we observed little or no improvements in standing, walking, running, or jumping ability as measured using the HFMSE; however, scores for items related to trunk control, such as lying, rolling, sitting, crawling, and kneeling improved following treatment [9]. In a previous study by Rosenblum et al., development of trunk control was identified as a prerequisite for upper extremity function and manual dexterity in healthy children [10]. Wang et al. also noted that development of trunk control in preterm infants improved fine motor skills [11]. This is because trunk stability plays an important role in upper limb motor function [12]. In accordance with previous findings, the improvements in PP score observed in this study are presumed to include the effect of improved trunk control, as measured using the HFMSE.

In addition, a recent study by Bram et al. showed significant improvements in hand grip strength and hand motor function in adult patients with SMA type 3 and 4 treated with nusinersen [5]. Similarly, administration of nusinersen may have improved fine motor function of the hand itself in our patients with SMA type 2.

In comparing the fine manual dexterity of SMA type 2 patients treated with nusinersen versus normal children, most SMA patients before receiving nusinersen had lower PP test scores than normal children of the same age and sex. However, the scores improved to the normal range observed from healthy children in most patients treated for 18 months (Figure 3) [8,13]. In a previous study, it was reported that when nusinersen was administered to infants during the pre-symptomatic stage, most patients achieved the motor milestone within the window for healthy children [14]. Similar to the results of the previous study, it is postulated that nusinersen administration rapidly improved fine manual dexterity in SMA patients; thus, they were able to reduce the gap with the normal fine motor milestone.

Previous studies have demonstrated that patients with SMA treated with nusinersen exhibit improvements not only in HFMSE scores but also in upper arm skill, as assessed using the RULM [4]. The RULM is designed to evaluate upper limb functions closely related to activities of daily living [15]. Although the RULM has the advantage of evaluating the overall function of the upper extremities, it has limitations in quantitatively measuring fine manual dexterity. Considering that most patients with SMA type 2 cannot stand alone or walk with assistance, even if they receive nusinersen treatment, fine manual dexterity is important for activities of daily living in these patients. Simply adding the PP test to the battery of existing evaluation tools may aid in providing a more detailed assessment of fine manual dexterity in patients with SMA.

Since this study was conducted only on patients with SMA type 2, the effect of nusinersen on fine manual dexterity in patients with other subtypes of SMA could not be identified. In a previous study, comparing the effects of nusinersen on SMA types 2 and 3, the change in the HFMSE score was greater in SMA type 2 than in SMA type 3 (+10.8 points versus +1.8 points) while the change in the upper limb module (ULM) score was also greater in SMA type 2 [16]. Considering the results of this previous study, it is presumed that the benefits of nusinersen on fine manual dexterity will also be greater in type 2 SMA than in other later-onset SMA types; however, this remains to be confirmed through further studies.

The present study had some limitations. Although nusinersen improved fine manual dexterity in a small number of subjects with SMA, this effect may not be statistically significant in large-scale studies. The statistical significance of the results of this study will be confirmed through a large multicenter study. Additionally, only the PP test was used to evaluate fine manual dexterity. Use of other tools to evaluate fine manual dexterity may have yielded more robust findings. Despite these limitations, this study is meaningful in that it is the first to report improvements in fine manual dexterity after nusinersen administration in patients with SMA type 2. Nonetheless, further studies including larger numbers of patients are required to verify our findings.

5. Conclusions

Changes in PP scores from baseline to 18 months confirmed that nusinersen treatment improved fine manual dexterity in patients with SMA type 2. Simply adding the PP test to the existing battery of evaluation tools may help to provide a more thorough assessment of the fine manual dexterity essential for daily living activities in patients with SMA type 2.

Author Contributions: Conceptualization, M.G. and H.-H.K.; methodology, H.-H.K.; software, M.G.; formal analysis, M.G. and H.-H.K.; investigation, H.-H.K.; resources, H.-H.K.; data curation, M.G.; writing—original draft preparation, M.G.; writing—review and editing, H.-H.K.; visualization, M.G.; supervision, H.-H.K. All authors have read and agreed to the published version of the manuscript.

Funding: This research received no external funding.

Institutional Review Board Statement: This study was approved by the Institutional Review Board of the Chungbuk National University (IRB number: CBNUH 2021-08-011, date of approval: 18 August 2021).

Informed Consent Statement: Patient consent was waived due to the type of study (retrospective, based on existing data).

Conflicts of Interest: The authors declare no conflict of interest.

References

1. Prasad, A.N.; Prasad, C.J.B. The floppy infant: Contribution of genetic and metabolic disorders. *Brain Dev.* **2003**, *25*, 457–476. [CrossRef]
2. Lefebvre, S.; Burglen, L.; Reboullet, S.; Clermont, O.; Burlet, P.; Viollet, L.; Benichou, B.; Cruaud, C.; Millasseau, P.; Zeviani, M.; et al. Identification and characterization of a spinal muscular atrophy-determining gene. *Cell* **1995**, *80*, 155–165. [CrossRef]
3. Iyer, C.C.; McGovern, V.L.; Murray, J.D.; Gombash, S.E.; Zaworski, P.G.; Foust, K.D.; Janssen, P.M.L.; Burghes, A.H.M. Low levels of Survival Motor Neuron protein are sufficient for normal muscle function in the SMNDelta7 mouse model of SMA. *Hum. Mol. Genet.* **2015**, *24*, 6160–6173. [CrossRef] [PubMed]
4. Mercuri, E.; Darras, B.T.; Chiriboga, C.A.; Day, J.W.; Campbell, C.; Connolly, A.M.; Iannaccone, S.T.; Kirschner, J.; Kuntz, N.; Saito, K.; et al. Nusinersen versus sham control in later-onset spinal muscular atrophy. *N. Engl. J. Med.* **2018**, *378*, 625–635. [CrossRef] [PubMed]

5. De Wel, B.; Goosens, V.; Sobota, A.; Camp, E.V.; Geukens, E.; Van Kerschaver, G.; Jagut, M.; Claes, K.; Claeys, K.G. Nusinersen treatment significantly improves hand grip strength, hand motor function and MRC sum scores in adult patients with spinal muscular atrophy types 3 and 4. *J. Neurol.* **2021**, *268*, 923–935. [CrossRef]
6. O'Hagen, J.M.; Glanzman, A.M.; McDermott, M.P.; Ryan, P.A.; Flickinger, J.; Quigely, J.; Riley, S.; Saborn, E.; Irvine, C.; Martens, W.B.; et al. An expanded version of the Hammersmith Functional Motor Scale for SMA II and III patients. *Neuromusc. Disord.* **2007**, *17*, 693–697. [CrossRef]
7. Glanzman, A.M.; O'Hagen, J.M.; McDermott, M.P.; Martens, W.B.; Flickinger, J.; Riley, S.; Quigely, J.; Montes, J.; Dunaway, S.; Deng, L.; et al. Validation of the Expanded Hammersmith Functional Motor Scale in spinal muscular atrophy type II and III. *J. Child Neurol.* **2011**, *26*, 1499–1507. [CrossRef] [PubMed]
8. Wilson, B.C.; Wilson, J.J.; Iacoviello, J.M.; Risucci, D. Purdue Pegboard performance of normal preschool children. *J. Clin. Neuropsychol.* **1982**, *4*, 19–26. [CrossRef] [PubMed]
9. Pin, T.W.; Butler, P.B.; Cheung, H.-M.; Shum, S.L.F. Relationship between segmental trunk control and gross motor development in typically developing infants aged from 4 to 12 months: A pilot study. *BMC Pediatr.* **2019**, *19*, 425. [CrossRef] [PubMed]
10. Rosenblum, S.; Josman, N.J.P. The relationship between postural control and fine manual dexterity. *Phys. Occup. Ther. Pediatr.* **2003**, *23*, 47–60. [CrossRef] [PubMed]
11. Wang, T.-N.; Howe, T.-H.; Hinojosa, J.; Weinberg, S.L. Relationship between postural control and fine motor skills in preterm infants at 6 and 12 months adjusted age. *Am. J. Occup. Ther.* **2011**, *65*, 695–701. [CrossRef] [PubMed]
12. Miyake, Y.; Kobayashi, R.; Kelepecz, D.; Nakajima, M. Core exercises elevate trunk stability to facilitate skilled motor behavior of the upper extremities. *J. Bodyw. Mov. Ther.* **2013**, *17*, 259–265. [CrossRef] [PubMed]
13. Gardner, R.A.; Broman, M. The Purdue Pegboard: Normative data on 1334 school children. *J. Clin. Child Psychol.* **1979**, *8*, 156–162. [CrossRef]
14. De Vivo, D.C.; Bertini, E.; Swoboda, K.J.; Hwu, W.L.; Crawford, T.O.; Finkel, R.S.; Kirschner, J.; Kuntz, N.L.; Parsons, J.A.; Ryan, M.M.; et al. Nusinersen initiated in infants during the presymptomatic stage of spinal muscular atrophy: Interim efficacy and safety results from the Phase 2 NURTURE study. *Neuromuscul. Disord.* **2019**, *29*, 842–856. [CrossRef] [PubMed]
15. Mazzone, E.S.; Mayhew, A.; Montes, J.; Ramsey, D.; Fanelli, L.; Dunaway Young, S.; Salazar, R.; De Sanctis, R.; Pasternak, A.; Glanzman, A.; et al. Revised upper limb module for spinal muscular atrophy: Development of a new module. *Muscle Nerve.* **2017**, *55*, 869–874. [CrossRef] [PubMed]
16. Darras, B.T.; Chiriboga, C.A.; Iannaccone, S.T.; Swoboda, K.J.; Montes, J.; Mignon, L.; Xia, S.; Bennett, C.F.; Bishop, K.M.; Shefner, J.M.; et al. Nusinersen in later-onset spinal muscular atrophy: Long-term results from the phase 1/2 studies. *Neurology.* **2019**, *92*, e2492–e2506. [CrossRef] [PubMed]

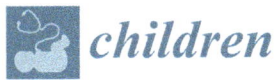

Article

Quality of Life Outcomes According to Differential Nusinersen Exposure in Pediatric Spinal Muscular Atrophy

Meaghann S. Weaver [1,2], Alice Yuroff [3], Sarah Sund [3], Scott Hetzel [3] and Matthew A. Halanski [1,*]

[1] Children's Hospital and Medical Center, Omaha, NE 68114, USA; meweaver@childrensomaha.org
[2] National Center for Ethics in Healthcare, Washington, DC 20420, USA
[3] School of Medicine and Public Health, University of Wisconsin-Madison, Madison, WI 53706, USA; Alice.Yuroff@fammed.wisc.edu (A.Y.); Sund@ortho.wisc.edu (S.S.); hetzel@biostat.wisc.edu (S.H.)
* Correspondence: mhalanski@childrensomaha.org; Tel.: +402-955-4160; Fax: +402-955-6330

Abstract: The purpose of this study was to explore early changes in patient and family caregiver report of quality of life and family impact during the transitional period of nusinersen use. Communication; family relationships; physical, emotional, social, and cognitive functioning; and daily activities were measured using Pediatric Quality of Life modules (Family Impact Modules and both Patient and Proxy Neuromuscular-Specific Reports) pre- and post-nusinersen exposure. A total of 35 patients with SMA (15 Type 1, 14 Type 2, and 6 Type 3) were grouped according to nusinersen exposure. When analyzed as a whole cross-sectional clinical population, no significant differences were found between the initial and final surveys. Nusinersen therapy was associated with improved communication and emotional functioning in subsets of the population, particularly for patients on maintenance therapy for longer duration. Several unexpected potentially negative findings including increases in family resources and trends towards increases in worry warrant further consideration. Further research is warranted to explore the impact of novel pharmaceuticals on quality of life for children with SMA longitudinally to optimize clinical and psychosocial outcomes.

Keywords: spinal muscular atrophy; quality of life; child neurology; patient-reported outcomes; neuromuscular

Citation: Weaver, M.S.; Yuroff, A.; Sund, S.; Hetzel, S.; Halanski, M.A. Quality of Life Outcomes According to Differential Nusinersen Exposure in Pediatric Spinal Muscular Atrophy. *Children* **2021**, *8*, 604. https://doi.org/10.3390/children8070604

Academic Editor: Rudolf Korinthenberg

Received: 15 June 2021
Accepted: 13 July 2021
Published: 17 July 2021

Publisher's Note: MDPI stays neutral with regard to jurisdictional claims in published maps and institutional affiliations.

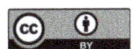

Copyright: © 2021 by the authors. Licensee MDPI, Basel, Switzerland. This article is an open access article distributed under the terms and conditions of the Creative Commons Attribution (CC BY) license (https://creativecommons.org/licenses/by/4.0/).

1. Introduction

Spinal muscular atrophy (SMA) is an autosomal-recessive, progressive neuromuscular disease associated with extensive morbidity related to muscular atrophy and proximal muscle weakness with risk for early mortality. In the past, children with SMA Type I seldom survived beyond the first few years of life even with mechanical respiratory support [1]. With the recent introduction of novel pharmaceutical interventions such as nusinersen [1,2] and gene therapies [3], children with SMA now have potentially increased lifespans and improved quality of life (QOL). A modified 2'-O-methoxyethyl antisense oligonucleotide by the name of nusinersen was approved by the Food and Drug Agency in December of 2016 with subsequent evidence of high efficacy and safety [4,5]. Quality of life outcomes associated with nusinersen use have been less studied.

A paucity of data exists on how children with SMA depict quality of life from their own report or how family caregivers of children with SMA perceive the diagnosis impacts the child and family before, during, and after the early phases of introducing nusinersen. As survival may be prolonged through medical advancements, learning about the child's QOL remains a compassionate, competent clinical care priority [6,7]. This knowledge can help clinicians partner with the child and family for symptom or support interventions intended to further support lived experiences. QOL is defined as "an individual's perception of his/her position in life in the context of culture and value systems in which he/she lives and in relation to wellness, goals, expectations, standards, and concerns" [8]. By investing in the subjective perspective of pediatric patients and their family caregivers before and after introduction of a therapy such as nusinersen, clinical teams are then positioned to better appreciate how therapies may trend with enhanced or burdened overall perceptions of health or wellness.

In 2016, prior to the widespread use of nusinersen at our institution, we began a study to evaluate the sensitivity of the Caregiver Priorities and Child Health Index of Life with Disabilities (CPCHILD™) questionnaire and PedsQL™ 3.0 Neuromuscular Module NMM (PedsQL) outcome measures to detect uniqueness between the between patient and proxy measurements and between SMA types [9]. We extended collection of the PedsQL outcome measures through 2019 to detect early changes in PEdsQL measurements in our clinical population during the transitional period of nusinersen use. This study highlights the early differences in PedsQL according to nusinersen exposure.

2. Materials and Methods

2.1. Participants and Setting

The University of Wisconsin-Madison Minimal Risk Institutional Review Board approved the study methodology and the ethics of implementation of this health sciences study in October 2015. Children and their family caregiver proxy were enrolled from November 2016 to September 2019. Eligibility criteria included patients with a diagnosis of SMA currently younger than age 18 receiving care at the outpatient neuromuscular clinic.

A letter was sent to eligible children/families providing details about the voluntary research study opportunity. The letter was mailed one to two weeks prior to the eligible subject's scheduled outpatient visit. The study coordinator then offered to meet with the patient and family caregiver through an informed consent process at the clinic visit. iPads linked wirelessly to the RedCAP© study database served as the survey response collection modality. The initial study included cross-over assessment of both the PedsQL™ 3.0 Neuromuscular Module (NMM) (for child-report and proxy-report) coupled with the PedsQL™ Family Impact Module (FIM) or CPCHILD™ questionnaire [9]. We continued collection of outcome measures until 2019 using the PedsQL measures as these appeared the most sensitive in our previous study in this population [9].

The electronic medical record was reviewed in a retrospective nature to determine the nusinersen status at the time of each initial questionnaire to produce four cohorts: (1) No Intent of Treatment, which included patients who did not start nor proceeded with any nusinesen treatment at time of final outcome measure; (2) Intent of Treatment, which included patients not on any treatment at time of initial questionnaire but began therapy after the initial assessment; (3) Loading Phase, which included patients within the first two months of treatment (received four intrathecal infusions) at the first quality of life (QOL) assessment; and (4) Maintenance Phase, which included patients on maintenance schedule (infusion every 4 months) at the time of initial QOL assessment. Cohorts 2–4 were receiving maintenance dosing at the time of their final survey (Figure 1). Pairwise differences between initial and final scores were analyzed within each cohort.

2.2. Methods

The PedsQL 3.0 Neuromuscular Module (NMM) includes 25 items covering core dimensions: (1) About My Neuromuscular Disease (17 items with emphasis on physical functioning), (2) Communication (3 items), and (3) About Our Family Resources (5 items). Child self-report and family proxy-reports are summarized for the past month. The PedsQL™ NMM maintains Cronbach's coefficient alpha scores >0.77 for each scale dimension in SMA cohorts [10–12].

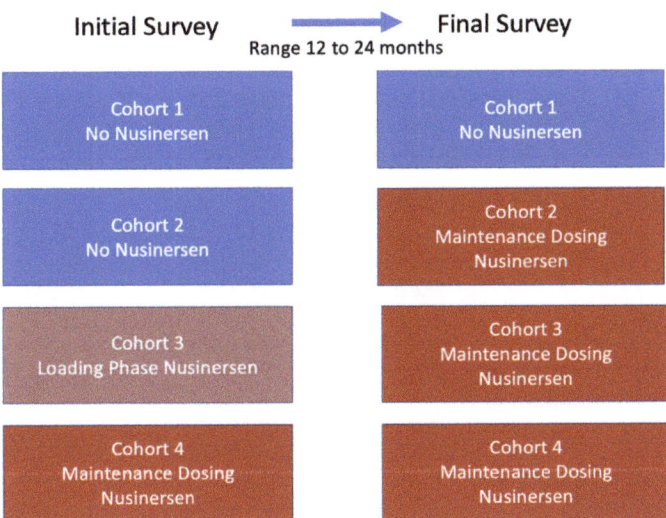

Figure 1. Nusinersen exposure at initial and final study timepoints. Legend—Transitions between nusinersen exposure during study initiation and follow-up timepoint including Cohort 1 which remained nusinersen naïve throughout; Cohort 2 which transitioned from no nusinersen to maintenance dosing; Cohort 3 which transitioned from loading phase to maintenance dosing; and Cohort 4 which remained on maintenance dosing with longest steady exposure to nusinersen.

The 36 item PedsQL Family Impact Module (FIM) measures parental perceptions of parental self-reported physical functioning (6 items), emotional functioning (5 items), social functioning (4 items), cognitive functioning (5 items), communication (3 items), and worry (5 items). The parent is reporting on his/her own well-being rather than the child's well-being over the past month. The PedsQL FIM explores the impact of the child's SMA diagnosis and neuromuscular health on family daily activities (3 items) and family relationships (5 items). In validation studies, Cronbach's coefficient alpha scores were >0.82 for PedsQL FIM scales [13].

2.3. Statistical Analysis

Survey total scores and sub-scores were calculated. Results were summarized using mean (SD) at each timepoint and the difference of means between the initial and final survey reported. Separate analyses were then performed based on SMA type or initial nusinersen status for those receiving nusinersen. Subjects in Cohorts 2 and 3 (no nusinersen at baseline and those in the loading phase) were also pooled together to assess any changes occurring once maintenance dosing is achieved. This combined cohort was then compared with those at on maintenance dosing at the time of initial survey. Comparisons of survey scores across two-level factors utilized t-tests, while comparisons of survey scores across three-level factors utilized ANOVA models. Due to the magnitude of testing, p-values were Benjamini–Hochberg corrected to control for false discovery rate [14]. Significant ANOVA p-values resulted in post hoc pairwise t-tests with Holm-adjusted p-values [15]. All tests had an adjusted alpha level of 0.05 and were conducted using R for Statistical Computing Version 3.5 [16].

3. Results

3.1. Participants

A total of 35 patients with SMA: 15 Type 1, 14 Type 2, and 6 Type 3, with a respective average age at initial survey (2.7+/−2.1), (11.2+/−5.9), (10.2+/−2.7) years and an average 1.8 (+/−0.5) years between surveys were analyzed. Five patients were in Cohort 1, the non-treatment control cohort containing two patients with Type 1, one patient with Type 2, and two patients with Type 3. Cohort 2 had $n = 8$ that had not started nusinersen at the time of the first survey, Cohort 3 had $n = 11$ that were in the loading phase of nusinersen at the time of the first survey, and Cohort 4 had $n = 11$ subjects already at the maintenance phase of treatment at the time of initial PedsQL. All patients in Cohorts 2–4 were on maintenance dosing at the time of the final QOL survey.

3.2. Collective Cohort

When analyzed as a whole cross-sectional clinical population (pooling Cohorts 2–4), no significant differences were found between the initial and final surveys for family impact (Table 1), child self-report (Table 2), or proxy family caregiver report (Table 3).

Table 1. PedsQL—Family Impact Module.

	Full Cohort ($n = 30$) *			
Variable	Baseline	Follow Up	Difference	p-Value
Physical Functioning	54.9 (21.8)	53.6 (20.5)	−1.2 (14.9)	0.65
Emotional Functioning	56.5 (21.5)	60.2 (20.6)	3.7 (14.2)	0.168
Social Functioning	50.4 (23.8)	50.6 (24.7)	0.2 (18.5)	0.951
Cognitive Functioning	56.2 (24.9)	59.6 (22.1)	3.3 (18.3)	0.326
Communication	50.3 (19.8)	54.2 (23.1)	3.9 (17.1)	0.222
Worry	51.3 (19.5)	55.7 (21.0)	4.3 (15.6)	0.138
Daily Activities	33.3 (23.1)	37.2 (29.4)	3.9 (21.9)	0.338
Family Relationship	60.0 (25.2)	63.7 (26.8)	3.7 (22.4)	0.377
PedsQL Family Impact Total Score	52.7 (18.9)	55.3 (19.5)	2.5 (11.0)	0.218
Parent HRQL Summary Score	54.6 (19.8)	56.0 (19.5)	1.3 (12.7)	0.574
Family Functioning Score	50.0 (22.3)	53.8 (26.5)	3.8 (19.6)	0.304

* Reported mean (SD); p-value from paired t-tests.

Table 2. Child Self-Repot PedsQL.

	Full Cohort ($n = 16$) *			
Variable	Baseline	Follow Up	Difference	p-Value
Neuromuscular Disease	56.7 (17.7)	56.2 (17.4)	−0.5 (12.0)	0.865
Communication	60.4 (40.4)	66.7 (30.5)	7.6 (23.4)	0.308
Family Resources	60.4 (25.7)	70.7 (18.0)	9.5 (18.0)	0.108
Total	58.2 (17.6)	59.9 (14.9)	1.7 (9.9)	0.497

* Reported as mean (SD); p-values are from paired t-tests.

Table 3. Proxy -Report (Family Caregiver) PedsQL.

	Full Cohort ($n = 30$) *			
Variable	Baseline	Follow Up	Difference	p-Value
Neuromuscular Disease	54.9 (16.5)	53.8 (15.7)	−1.1 (12.1)	0.625
Communication	43.9 (38.1)	48.1 (37.1)	4.2 (17.5)	0.202
Family Resources	50.8 (22.7)	55.3 (18.8)	4.5 (17.1)	0.16
Total	52.7 (17.4)	53.3 (16.2)	0.6 (10.6)	0.755

* Reported as mean (SD); p-values are from paired t-tests.

After sub-analyzing the data by SMA type and cohort (nusinersen status at the initial survey), several significant differences and trends were identified (Tables 4 and 5). In the Family Impact Module, improvements in emotional functioning were observed for children ($n = 8$) that progressed from no treatment to maintenance therapy (56.2+/−7.5→65.4+/−15.3, $p = 0.014$).

Table 4. Significant Difference in Quality of Life Scales by Cohort.

Module	Domain	Cohort	Baseline	Follow Up	Difference	p-Value
Child-PedsQL	Worry	SMA 1, n = 2	36.7 (15.3)	71.2 (11.8)	31.7 (2.9)	0.003
Child-PedsQL	Total Quality of Life	SMA 3, n = 3	68.4 (13.1)	73.0 (12.8)	4.6 (2.2)	0.068
Parent-PedsQL	Communication	SMA 3, n = 4	52.1 (25.8)	64.6 (31.5)	12.5 (8.3)	0.058
Parent-PedsQL	Family Resources	SMA 3, n = 4	58.8 (12.5)	68.8 (15.5)	10.0 (7.1)	0.066
Family Impact	Worry	SMA 1, n = 13	45.0 (12.7)	50.8 (12.6)	5.8 (9.8)	0.054
Family Impact	Daily Activities	SMA 2, n = 13	39.1 (28.1)	52.6 (32.5)	13.5 (23.9)	0.065

SMA 1, 2, and 3 reflect diagnostic subtype. colors are useful to reveal statistical significance reached vs. close.

Table 5. Significant Difference in Quality of Life Scales by Timeframe.

Module	Domain	Cohort	Baseline	Follow Up	Difference	p-Value
Child-PedsQL	Family Resources	L-M, n = 7	52.5 (26.4)	71.7 (15.4)	23.0 (12.5)	0.015
Parent-PedsQL	Communication	0 or L, n = 19	45.2 (34.5)	53.9 (33.7)	8.8 (17.2)	0.04
Parent-PedsQL	Communication	0-M, n = 8	53.1 (34.5)	67.7 (32.6)	14.6 (20.8)	0.087
Parent-PedsQL	Communication	M-M, n = 11	37.9 (42.1)	−3.8 (15.5)	0.437	0.056
Family Impact	Emotional Functioning	0 or L, n = 19	60.0 (16.2)	64.7 (15.6)	4.7 (9.9)	0.052
Family Impact	Emotional Functioning	0-M, n = 8	56.2 (7.5)	65.4 (15.3)	7.5 (2.9)	0.014
Family Impact	Emotional Functioning	M-M, n = 11	53.0 (16.7)	57.1 (28.5)	8.0 (12.7)	0.078
Family Impact	Communication	0-M, n = 8	54.2 (10.8)	55.6 (26.7)	8.3 (6.8)	0.092
Family Impact	Communication	M-M, n = 11	43.3 (19.6)	54.2 (25.0)	13.3 (17.7)	0.041
Family Impact	Worry	M-M, n = 11	44.5 (16.1)	57.9 (23.2)	10.5 (15.2)	0.056
Family Impact	HRQL Summary Score	M-M, n = 11	47.0 (12.2)	52.7 (26.6)	7.2 (11.6)	0.08
Family Impact	Family Impact Total Score	M-M, n = 11	45.7 (13.0)	52.4 (26.1)	8.6 (10.2)	0.027

Abbreviations—0 = No Nusinersen, L = Loading Phase, and M = Maintenance Dosing.

Patients on the maintenance dosing at the time of the initial questionnaire and therefore on maintenance therapy for longer duration (increased time exposure to nusinersen) demonstrated significant improvements in communication (43.3+/−19.6→54.2+/−25, $p = 0.041$). Per the Parental-PedsQL, improvements in communication trended towards improvement in patients initiating therapy and reaching maintenance dosing (Cohort 2) (53.1 +/−34.5→67.7+/−32.6, $p = 0.089$) and became significant when pooled with Cohort 3 (45.2+/−34.5→53.9+/−33.7, $p = 0.04$) demonstrating an improvement in communication scores when maintenance dosing was achieved and sustained.

Improvements in daily activities (39.1+/−28.1→52.6+/−32.5, $p = 0.065$) and PedsQL Family Impact Total Score (59.2+/−21.2→64.2+/−21.8, $p = 0.081$) domains trended towards significance in the population with SMA Type 2.

Patients on the maintenance dosing at the time of the initial questionnaire (again, with increased time exposure to nusinersen) demonstrated significant improvements in PedsQL Family Impact Total Score (45.7+/−13→52.6+/−26.1; $p = 0.027$).

While the majority of findings demonstrated improvements for the patents and families undergoing nusinersen treatment, several unaccepted adverse findings became apparent. First, the Family Resources Domain in the Child-PedsQL (N = 4) was significantly higher at follow up in the SMA Type 1 cohort (36.7+/−15.3→71.2+/−31.7, $p = 0.003$) and appeared to most affect those progressing from the loading to the maintenance phase (52.5+/−26→71.7+/−15.4; $p = 0.015$) (N = 7) and trended similarly in the Parental-PedsQL for patients with SMA Type 3 (58.8+/−12.5→68.8+/−15.5, $p = 0.066$).

Increases in the Worry domain also trended towards significance in our Family Impact Module for the SMA Type 1 cohort (45+/−12.7→50.8+/−12.6; $p = 0.054$) and surprisingly for those on the maintenance dosing for the entirety of this study (Cohort 4) 44.5+/−16.1→57.9+/−23.2, $p = 0.056$.

4. Discussion

In the PedsQL scale, a change of 5 in the Standard Error of the Mean (SEM) has been pre-determined to represent a minimally clinically important difference [17,18]. Thus, while noted change did not reach statistical significant difference when the at-large group was analyzed, MCID was reached for communication and family resources according to child self-report.

The major domains impacted during nusinersen treatment between the no treatment cohort and all SMA types were communication and emotional functioning. The major domain impacted during nusinersen treatment between SMA Type 1 and other SMA types was worry. Of interest, improvements in daily activities and Family Impact total score were significant only in patients with SMA Type 2. This may be due to the number of patients with Type 2 included in this study or may be due to other factors since there was no difference observed in baseline and follow up. Prior analyses by SMA type have revealed benefits in axial, proximal, and distal motor function, particularly for those with more severe forms of the disorder [3,4].

In this cross-sectional clinical study, utilizing patient reported outcome measures validated in the SMA population, nusinersen therapy was found to improve communication and emotional functioning in subsets of the population. However, several unexpected potentially negative findings including increases in family resources and trends towards increases in worry (particularly in those on the medication for the longest period of time) warrant further consideration.

4.1. Improvement in Communication and Emotional Functioning

This study revealed the benefits of nusinersen on psychosocial function beyond physiologic metrics, recognizing the importance of family communication for starting the medication and in goal setting for sustaining the medication. Nusinersen has been shown to prolong survival in infants with SMA [19–22] and improve motor function [23,24] and yet the impact of treatment options on family-based communication quality and satisfaction has been under-explored. The PedsQL FIM specifically asks about the experience of the family in communicating with the child's doctors and nurses about how they feel in addition to questions about communicating with friends and other extended family members. In a qualitative study of 19 parents engaged in decision making for their children with SMA, the most important factor for parental decision making was "honest communication with physicians" [25]. For parents in Germany whose children received nusinersen via an expanded access program, "good communication and trusting relationships with medical and non-medical staff at the hospital helped caregivers cope with the uncertainties associated with the treatment" [26]. Fifty-one parents of Swedish children with SMA emphasized the desire for health care professionals to not only possess knowledge but to provide knowledge [27], seemingly as a means to foster family communication and concordance in family decision making.

A population-based study among 34 Danish parents of children with severe SMA revealed the prioritized importance parents place on provider communication that specifies what SMA entails, the treatment options, and prognosis [28]. Among 95 parents of children with severe SMA in Denmark and Sweden, bereaved parents were significantly more satisfied with care than non-bereaved parents (81% vs. 29%), with noted emphasis on communication as part of care coordination [29].

While medical outcomes matter, families also highly regard and uphold the process of communication as formative in their family experience. Introducing nusinersen as a treatment option necessarily results in engagement about current and anticipated research findings, potential benefits and harms, and experiences of other families. This treatment-dialogue has potential to improve knowledge and empower communication within families.

4.2. Increase in Use of Family Resources

This study revealed that use of family resources was perceived as significantly increased for children with Type 1 SMA receiving nusinersen according to child self-report. Parents in this study did not document parallel perception of increased use of family resources according. This speaks to the pediatric patient's awareness of the investment of family time and finances to nusinersen as a biomedical intervention. The ways in which children with complex care needs may internally compare their resource requirements as compared to healthy peers or siblings, and how this translates into a child's sense of self (whether the child views herself as worthy or as burdensome) or perception of stress (whether the child carries undue fear about fiscal wellness for others in the family) have been under-explored and even under-recognized by health systems. Parents in this study may have normalized resource utilization out of deep regard for their child's access to the intervention and inability to place a resource measure on the infinite value of their child's life.

Parents of children starting nusinersen describe striving for longer duration of life and improved quality of life [30] in the setting of invasive treatment and complex care with frequent hospital-based procedures. Parents of children with SMA starting nusinersen have reported worries about the high cost and maintaining adequate insurance coverage; potential side effects, risk factors, and adverse events; and treatment time [31]. The indirect care coverage costs and foregone parental employment add to the direct medical costs along with the hidden cost of mental health strain [32]. In a study of 64 parents of children with SMA, family finances were depicted as an under-recognized and yet realistic family concern [33]. In a study of parents of children w/ SMA Types 2 and 3 in Australia, parents described: "significant financial and caregiving burdens, adjusted career choices and limitations on career progression and a complex landscape of access to funding, equipment, support and resources" [32].

From a health system perspective, the average annual cost of SMA1 "ranged from $75,047 to $196,429 per year" [34]. The "incremental cost-effectiveness ratio (ICER) of nusinersen compared to standard of care in SMA1 ranged from $210,095 to $1,150,455 per quality-adjusted life years (QALY) gained." [34] In a health resource comparison study, patients in the SMA Type I group ($n = 349$) and SMA Type 1 nusineran group ($n = 45$) "experienced an average of 59.4 and 56.6 days with medical visits per-patient-per-year (PPPY), respectively, including 14.1 and 4.6 inpatient days." [35] Regardless of pharmaceutical or hospital-use economic impact, families of children receiving motor, speech, and survival benefit from nusinersen speak of the miraculous impact of the medication, which exceeds a describable cost value for those children and families.

4.3. Increase in Worry

An important finding from this study was how worry started at the lowest in the maintenance cohort, but worry notably increased longitudinally. Prior studies have shown worry peak at time of decision making about starting a new medication with unknown outcomes and concern for side effects. While nusinersen has been shown to prolong survival in infants with SMA [19–22] and improve motor function [23,24], the parents involved in this study engaged in treatment decision making prior to the more recent accumulation of outcomes-based data and thus were venturing into the unknown.

Guilt regarding genetic diagnoses and uncertainties introduced by new therapies compound the underlying unpredictable trajectory of SMA [36,37], resulting in realistic worry at medication start. Parents of children starting nusinersen report worrying about "making difficult treatment choices" as well as "reactions, side effects, and worsening quality of life" [33,38]. A qualitative study of German parents of children with SMA Type 1 depicted "significant uncertainty and stress among caregivers prior to the actual treatment. Further, concerns persisted that nusinersen could not be approved or that the child could be excluded due to an insufficient treatment response" [26]. While medical teams may consider nusinersen generally well tolerated and efficacious, parents depict worry about their child not responding to nusinersen, requiring treatment interruptions, and experiencing complications [39].

As data show that earlier initiation of treatment is associated with more efficacy on functionality (such as ambulation) [40], family caregivers recognize time-sensitive decision making which may compound the sense of worry or urgency at initiation. Secondary spine and thorax deformities are frequent in children with SMA [41], adding worry for many families about not only the frequency of sedation but also the lumbar puncture itself [42]. Parents weigh the hoped-for benefits of nusinersen with concern about the child's discomfort. Even for parents of children with SMA who did not experience nusinersen-related adverse events, realities of disease-specific adverse events such as cough, respiratory infections, and weakness continue to cause concern [4]. This study revealed that worry did not dissolve or mitigate with time, but instead seemed to increase longitudinally. This pattern of sustained worry as captured in this study hints at ongoing concern that patients and families have about whether the medication will continue working, whether there will be a delayed side effect, and the extent to which benefit may be sustained.

4.4. Study Strengths and Limitations

Strengths of this study include access to not only proxy-report but also pediatric patient-reported outcomes, now recognized as the gold standard for drug impact reporting [43]. Additional study strength includes use of quality of life metrics validated for this population and obtainment of surveys at more than one timepoint. Study limitations include single-site enrollment. This study did not control for whether children had missed any doses of nusinersen or adverse event/side effect profile of medication administration.

5. Conclusions

Nusinersen has offered a form of medical hope to children with SMA and their family caregivers with measurable impact on motor function and ambulation, despite the cost and challenges with administration. As the science advances to now include gene therapy, an interim goal would be additional treatment options with less burden on patients for SMA such as oral administration or one-time infusions. The lived experience of children with SMA receiving nusinersen warrants attentiveness towards ways to continually improve their quality of life. This includes consideration of ways to support family emotion and economic burden as well as foster family-centric communication. Future studies would ideally explore the impact of nusinersen and novel pharmaceutical interventions on functional abilities chronologically and longitudinally with correlated quality of life and family impact metrics.

Author Contributions: Conceptualization, A.Y., S.S. and M.A.H.; methodology, A.Y., S.S. and M.A.H.; software, S.H.; formal analysis, S.H.; investigation, M.S.W., A.Y., S.S., S.H. and M.A.H.; data curation, A.Y., S.S., S.H. and M.A.H. writing—original draft preparation, M.S.W. and M.A.H.; writing—review and editing, A.Y. and M.A.H.; supervision, M.A.H.; project administration, S.S. All authors have read and agreed to the published version of the manuscript.

Funding: The authors would like to acknowledge support from the UW-ICTR PCORI Pilot Program.

Institutional Review Board Statement: This study was conducted according to the guidelines of the Declaration of Helsinki, and approved by the local Institutional Review Board. The committee name is University of Wisconsin—Madison Minimal Risk IRB (Health Sciences). The ID for this study is 2015-1039. Initial Approval: 10 December 2015.

Informed Consent Statement: Informed consent and/or assent (age-dependent) was obtained from all subjects involved in this study.

Data Availability Statement: Data can be made available upon reasonable request to senior author.

Acknowledgments: Gratitude to the patients and families involved in this study. The authors would like to acknowledge support from the UW-ICTR PCORI Pilot Program.

Conflicts of Interest: The authors declare no conflict of interest. Weaver contributed to this paper in a private capacity. No official support or endorsement by the U.S. Department of Veterans Affairs is intended, nor should be inferred.

References

1. Pechmann, A.; Kirschner, J. Diagnosis and New Treatment Avenues in Spinal Muscular Atrophy. *Neuropediatrics* **2017**, *48*, 273–281. [CrossRef] [PubMed]
2. Ohmura, T.; Saeki, S.; Ogiwara, K.; Tobita, K.; Ling, Y.; Torii, S. Pharmacological and clinical profile of spinal muscular atrophy (SMA) therapeutic drug nusinersen (Spinraza(R)). *Nihon Yakurigaku Zasshi* **2018**, *152*, 147–159. [CrossRef]
3. Messina, S.; Sframeli, M.; Maggi, L.; D'Amico, A.; Bruno, C.; Comi, G.; Mercuri, E. Spinal muscular atrophy: State of the art and new therapeutic strategies. *Neurol. Sci.* **2021**, 1–10. [CrossRef]
4. Acsadi, G.; Crawford, T.O.; Muller-Felber, W.; Shieh, P.B.; Richardson, R.; Natarajan, N.; Castro, D.; Ramirez-Schrempp, D.; Gambino, G.; Sun, P.; et al. Safety and efficacy of nusinersen in spinal muscular atrophy: The EMBRACE study. *Muscle Nerve* **2021**, *63*, 668–677. [CrossRef] [PubMed]
5. De Vivo, D.C.; Bertini, E.; Swoboda, K.J.; Hwu, W.-L.; Crawford, T.O.; Finkel, R.S.; Kirschner, J.; Kuntz, N.L.; Parsons, J.A.; Ryan, M.M.; et al. Nusinersen initiated in infants during the presymptomatic stage of spinal muscular atrophy: Interim efficacy and safety results from the Phase 2 NURTURE study. *Neuromuscul Disord.* **2019**, *29*, 842–856. [CrossRef] [PubMed]
6. Lovgren, M.; Sejersen, T.; Kreicbergs, U. Parents' Experiences and Wishes at End of Life in Children with Spinal Muscular Atrophy Types I and II. *J. Pediatr.* **2016**, *175*, 201–205. [CrossRef] [PubMed]
7. Lovgren, M.; Sejersen, T.; Kreicbergs, U. Information and treatment decisions in severe spinal muscular atrophy: A parental follow-up. *Eur. J. Paediatr. Neurol.* **2016**, *20*, 830–838. [CrossRef] [PubMed]
8. Khanna, D.; Tsevat, J. Health-related quality of life–an introduction. *Am. J. Manag. Care* **2007**, *13* (Suppl. 9), S218–S223.
9. Weaver, M.S.; Hanna, R.; Hetzel, S.; Patterson, K.; Yuroff, A.; Sund, S.; Schultz, M.; Schroth, M.; Halanski, M.A. A Prospective, Crossover Survey Study of Child- and Proxy-Reported Quality of Life According to Spinal Muscular Atrophy Type and Medical Interventions. *J. Child Neurol.* **2020**, *35*, 322–330. [CrossRef]
10. Klug, C.; Schreiber-Katz, O.; Thiele, S.; Schorling, E.; Zowe, J.; Reilich, P.; Walter, M.C.; Nagels, K.H. Disease burden of spinal muscular atrophy in Germany. *Orphanet J. Rare Dis.* **2016**, *11*, 58. [CrossRef]
11. Iannaccone, S.T.; Hynan, L.S.; Morton, A.; Buchanan, R.; Limbers, C.A.; Varni, J.W.; AmSMART Group. The PedsQL in pediatric patients with Spinal Muscular Atrophy: Feasibility, reliability, and validity of the Pediatric Quality of Life Inventory Generic Core Scales and Neuromuscular Module. *Neuromuscul Disord.* **2009**, *19*, 805–812. [CrossRef] [PubMed]
12. Kocova, H.; Dvorackova, O.; Vondracek, P.; Haberlova, J. Health-related quality of life in children and adolescents with spinal muscular atrophy in the Czech Republic. *Pediatric Neurol.* **2014**, *50*, 591–594. [CrossRef]
13. Varni, J.W.; Sherman, S.A.; Burwinkle, T.M.; Dickinson, P.E.; Dixon, P. The PedsQL Family Impact Module: Preliminary reliability and validity. *Health Qual. Life Outcomes* **2004**, *2*, 55. [CrossRef]
14. Benjamini, Y.; Hochberg, Y. Controlling the False Discovery Rate: A Practical and Powerful Approach to Multiple Testing. *J. R. Stat. Soc. Ser. B Methodol.* **1995**, *57*, 289–300. [CrossRef]
15. Holm, S. A simple sequentially rejective multiple test procedure. *Scand. J. Stat.* **1979**, *6*, 65–70.
16. Team RC. A language and environment for statistical computing. Available online: https://www.R-project.org/ (accessed on 24 May 2019).
17. Norman, G.R.; Sloan, J.A.; Wyrwich, K.W. Interpretation of changes in health-related quality of life: The remarkable universality of half a standard deviation. *Med. Care* **2003**, *41*, 582–592. [CrossRef]
18. Weaver, M.; Wichman, C.; Darnall, C.; Bace, S.; Vail, C.; MacFadyen, A. Proxy-Reported Quality of Life and Family Impact for Children Followed Longitudinally by a Pediatric Palliative Care Team. *J. Palliat. Med.* **2018**, *21*, 241–244. [CrossRef] [PubMed]
19. Chiriboga, C.A.; Swoboda, K.J.; Darras, B.T.; Iannaccone, S.T.; Montes, J.; De Vivo, D.C.; Norris, D.A.; Bennett, C.F.; Bishop, K.M. Results from a phase 1 study of nusinersen (ISIS-SMN(Rx)) in children with spinal muscular atrophy. *Neurology* **2016**, *86*, 890–897. [CrossRef]
20. Finkel, R.S.; Chiriboga, C.A.; Vajsar, J.; Day, J.W.; Montes, J.; De Vivo, D.C.; Bishop, K.M.; Foster, R.; Liu, Y.; Ramirez-Schrempp, D.; et al. Treatment of infantile-onset spinal muscular atrophy with nusinersen: A phase 2, open-label, dose-escalation study. *Lancet* **2016**, *388*, 3017–3026. [CrossRef]
21. Finkel, R.S.; Mercuri, E.; Darras, B.T.; Connolly, A.M.; Kuntz, N.L.; Kirschner, J.; Chiriboga, C.A.; Saito, K.; Servais, L.; Tizzano, E.; et al. Nusinersen versus Sham Control in Infantile-Onset Spinal Muscular Atrophy. *N. Engl. J. Med.* **2017**, *377*, 1723–1732. [CrossRef]
22. Mercuri, E.; Darras, B.T.; Chiriboga, C.A.; Day, J.W.; Campbell, C.; Connolly, A.M.; Iannaccone, S.T.; Kirschner, J.; Kuntz, N.L.; Saito, K.; et al. Nusinersen versus Sham Control in Later-Onset Spinal Muscular Atrophy. *N. Engl. J. Med.* **2018**, *378*, 625–635. [CrossRef]
23. Pane, M.; Coratti, G.; Sansone, V.A.; Messina, S.; Catteruccia, M.; Bruno, C.; Sframeli, M.; Albamonte, E.; Pedemonte, M.; D'Amico, A.; et al. Italian EAP Working Group. Type I SMA new natural history: Long-term data in nusinersen-treated patients. *Ann. Clin. Transl. Neurol.* **2021**, *8*, 548–557. [CrossRef]
24. Osredkar, D.; Jilkova, M.; Butenko, T.; Loboda, T.; Golli, T.; Fuchsová, P.; Rohlenová, M.; Haberlova, J. Children and young adults with spinal muscular atrophy treated with nusinersen. *Eur. J. Paediatr. Neurol.* **2020**, *30*, 1–8. [CrossRef]
25. van Kruijsbergen, M.; Schroder, C.D.; Ketelaar, M.; van der Pol, W.; Cuppen, I.; van deer Geest, A.; Asselman, F.-L.; Fischer, M.J.; Vissert-Meily, J.M.A.; Kars, M.C. Parents' perspectives on nusinersen treatment for children with spinal muscular atrophy. *Dev. Med. Child Neurol.* **2021**, *63*, 816–823. [CrossRef]

26. Kiefer, P.; Kirschner, J.; Pechmann, A.; Langer, T. Experiences of caregivers of children with spinal muscular atrophy participating in the expanded access program for nusinersen: A longitudinal qualitative study. *Orphanet J. Rare Dis.* **2020**, *15*, 194. [CrossRef]
27. Hjorth, E.; Kreicbergs, U.; Sejersen, T.; Lovgren, M. Parents' advice to healthcare professionals working with children who have spinal muscular atrophy. *Eur. J. Paediatr. Neurol.* **2018**, *22*, 128–134. [CrossRef] [PubMed]
28. Beernaert, K.; Lovgren, M.; Jeppesen, J.; Werlauff, U.; Rahbek, J.; Sejersen, T.; Kreicbergs, U. Parents' Experiences of Information and Decision Making in the Care of Their Child With Severe Spinal Muscular Atrophy: A Population Survey. *J. Child Neurol.* **2019**, *34*, 210–215. [CrossRef]
29. Hjorth, E.; Kreicbergs, U.; Sejersen, T.; Jeppesen, J.; Werlauffm, U.; Rahbek, J.; Lövgren, M. Bereaved Parents More Satisfied With the Care Given to Their Child With Severe Spinal Muscular Atrophy Than Nonbereaved. *J. Child Neurol.* **2019**, *34*, 104–112. [CrossRef]
30. Benini, F.; Salamon, E.; Divisic, A.; Maghini, I.; Agosto, C. Acknowledging Limits: Statistics and the Child's Quality of Life in Spinal Muscular Atrophy. *J. Paediatr. Child Health* **2020**, *56*, 995–996. [CrossRef] [PubMed]
31. Pacione, M.; Siskind, C.E.; Day, J.W.; Tabor, H.K. Perspectives on Spinraza (Nusinersen) Treatment Study: Views of Individuals and Parents of Children Diagnosed with Spinal Muscular Atrophy. *J. Neuromuscul Dis.* **2019**, *6*, 119–131. [CrossRef] [PubMed]
32. Farrar, M.A.; Carey, K.A.; Paguinto, S.G.; Chambers, G.; Kasparian, N.A. Financial, opportunity and psychosocial costs of spinal muscular atrophy: An exploratory qualitative analysis of Australian carer perspectives. *BMJ Open* **2018**, *8*, e020907. [CrossRef]
33. Qian, Y.; McGraw, S.; Henne, J.; Jarecki, J.; Hobby, K.; Yeh, W.S. Understanding the experiences and needs of individuals with Spinal Muscular Atrophy and their parents: A qualitative study. *BMC Neurol.* **2015**, *15*, 217. [CrossRef] [PubMed]
34. Dangouloff, T.; Botty, C.; Beaudart, C.; Servais, L.; Hiligsmann, M. Systematic literature review of the economic burden of spinal muscular atrophy and economic evaluations of treatments. *Orphanet J. Rare Dis.* **2021**, *16*, 47. [CrossRef] [PubMed]
35. Droege, M.; Sproule, D.; Arjunji, R.; Gauthier-Loiselle, M.; Cloutier, M.; Dabbous, O. Economic burden of spinal muscular atrophy in the United States: A contemporary assessment. *J. Med. Econ.* **2020**, *23*, 70–79. [CrossRef]
36. James, C.A.; Hadley, D.W.; Holtzman, N.A.; Winkelstein, J.A. How does the mode of inheritance of a genetic condition influence families? A study of guilt, blame, stigma, and understanding of inheritance and reproductive risks in families with X-linked and autosomal recessive diseases. *Genet. Med.* **2006**, *8*, 234–242. [CrossRef]
37. Arribas-Ayllon, M.; Sarangi, S.; Clarke, A. Managing self-responsibility through other-oriented blame: Family accounts of genetic testing. *Soc. Sci. Med.* **2008**, *66*, 1521–1532. [CrossRef] [PubMed]
38. Cruz, R.; Belter, L.; Wasnock, M.; Nazarelli, A.; Jarecki, J. Evaluating Benefit-risk Decision-making in Spinal Muscular Atrophy: A First-ever Study to Assess Risk Tolerance in the SMA Patient Community. *Clin. Ther.* **2019**, *41*, 943–960. [CrossRef] [PubMed]
39. Agosto, C.; Salamon, E.; Divisic, A.; Benedetti, F.; Giacomelli, L.; Shah, A.; Perilongo, G.; Benini, F. Do we always need to treat patients with spinal muscular atrophy? A personal view and experience. *Orphanet J. Rare Dis.* **2021**, *16*, 78. [CrossRef]
40. Audic, F.; de la Banda, M.G.G.; Bernoux, D.; Ramirez-Garcia, P.; Durigneux, J.; Barnerias, C.; Isapof, A.; Cuisset, J.; Cances, C.; Richelme, C.; et al. Effects of nusinersen after one year of treatment in 123 children with SMA type 1 or 2: A French real-life observational study. *Orphanet J. Rare Dis.* **2020**, *15*, 148. [CrossRef]
41. Johannsen, J.; Weiss, D.; Schlenker, F.; Groth, M.; Denecke, J. Intrathecal Administration of Nusinersen in Pediatric SMA Patients with and without Spine Deformities: Experiences and Challenges over 3 Years in a Single Center. *Neuropediatrics* **2020**, *52*, 179–185. [CrossRef]
42. Goedeker, N.L.; Gibbons, J.L.; Varadhachary, A.S.; Connolly, A.M.; Zaidman, C.M. Laboratory Monitoring of Nusinersen Safety. *Muscle Nerve* **2021**, *63*, 902–905. [CrossRef] [PubMed]
43. Leahy, A.B.; Steineck, A. Patient-Reported Outcomes in Pediatric Oncology: The Patient Voice as a Gold Standard. *JAMA Pediatrics* **2020**, *174*, e202868. [CrossRef] [PubMed]

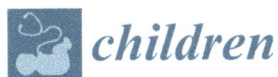

Article

Sagittal Plane Deformities in Children with SMA2 following Posterior Spinal Instrumentation

Matthew A. Halanski [1], Rewais Hanna [2], James Bernatz [2], Max Twedt [1], Sarah Sund [2], Karen Patterson [2], Kenneth J. Noonan [2], Meredith Schultz [3], Mary K. Schroth [4], Mark Sharafinski [2] and Brian P. Hasley [1,*]

[1] Department of Orthopaedic Surgery, University of Nebraska Medical Center, Omaha, NE 68198, USA; mhalanski@childrensomaha.org (M.A.H.); max.twedt@unmc.edu (M.T.)
[2] School of Medicine and Public Health, University of Wisconsin-Madison, Madison, WI 53706, USA; rbhanna@wisc.edu (R.H.); JBernatz@uwhealth.org (J.B.); Sund@ortho.wisc.edu (S.S.); pattersonk@pt.wisc.edu (K.P.); Noonan@ortho.wisc.edu (K.J.N.); msharafinski@uwhealth.org (M.S.)
[3] Novartis Gene Therapies, 2275 Half Day Road, Suite 200, Bannockburn, IL 60015, USA; mschultz465@avexis.com
[4] Cure SMA, 925 Busse Road, Elk Grove Village, IL 60007, USA; mary@curesma.org
* Correspondence: brhasley@childrensomaha.org; Tel.: +1-(402)-955-6317

Abstract: This is a retrospective radiographic review to assess post-operative sagittal plane deformities in patients with Spinal Muscular Atrophy type 2 that had been treated with posterior spinal instrumentation. Thirty-two patients with a history of either spinal fusion (N = 20) or growing rods (N = 12) were identified with an average of 7.6 (2.1–16.6) years post-operative follow-up. Forty percent (13/32) of the patients were identified as having obvious "tucked chin" (N = 4), "tipped trunk" (N = 9), or both (N = 3). Sacral incidence was the only parameter that was statistically significant change between pre-operative or immediate post-operative measurements (66.9° vs. 55.2° $p = 0.03$). However, at final follow-up, the post-operative thoracic kyphosis had decreased over time in those that developed a subsequent sagittal deformity (24.2°) whereas it increased in those that did not (44.7°, $p = 0.008$). This decrease in thoracic kyphosis throughout the instrumented levels, resulted in a greater lordotic imbalance (30.4° vs. 5.6°, $p = 0.001$) throughout the instrumented levels in the group that developed the subsequent cervical or pelvic sagittal deformities. In conclusion, sagittal plane deformities commonly develop outside the instrumented levels in children with SMA type 2 following posterior spinal instrumentation and may be the result of lordotic imbalance that occurs through continued anterior growth following posterior instrumentation.

Keywords: spinal muscular atrophy; posterior spinal fusion; kyphosis; sagittal plane deformity

Citation: Halanski, M.A.; Hanna, R.; Bernatz, J.; Twedt, M.; Sund, S.; Patterson, K.; Noonan, K.J.; Schultz, M.; Schroth, M.K.; Sharafinski, M.; et al. Sagittal Plane Deformities in Children with SMA2 following Posterior Spinal Instrumentation. *Children* 2021, 8, 703. https://doi.org/10.3390/children8080703

Academic Editor: Rudolf Korinthenberg

Received: 1 July 2021
Accepted: 2 August 2021
Published: 16 August 2021

Publisher's Note: MDPI stays neutral with regard to jurisdictional claims in published maps and institutional affiliations.

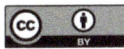

Copyright: © 2021 by the authors. Licensee MDPI, Basel, Switzerland. This article is an open access article distributed under the terms and conditions of the Creative Commons Attribution (CC BY) license (https://creativecommons.org/licenses/by/4.0/).

1. Introduction

Spinal Muscular Atrophy (SMA) is the most common fatal genetic disease affecting the pediatric population (1 in 6–10,000 live births). Classically, before the widespread use of disease modifying agents, children with this disease experienced progressive weakness and early mortality. SMA is classified into three types based on the onset of disease: type 1 has symptoms starting before 6 months of age, type 2 has onset between 6–18 months of age, and type 3 has onset after 18 months of age [1]. Children with type 1 never sit and without intervention have a life expectancy <2 years, type 2 sit but do not walk and survive into the second decade, and type 3 ambulate and have a life expectancy into adulthood [1]. Respiratory failure is the most frequent cause of death in children with SMA type 1 or 2 [2].

Our institutional experience in treating severely affected children with SMA (types 1 and 2) [3–9] with spinal deformities [10,11] has led to clinical observations that a sub-set of children with SMA type 2 (upright wheelchair sitters) developed very characteristic sagittal plane deformities following spinal instrumentation that resulted in either: (1) a "tipped trunk" deformity, in which the entire (fused) and unsupported trunk leans forward causing the abdomen to rest on the anterior thighs in the sitting position, resulting in a very prominent buttock posteriorly that complicates seating support of the lumbar and thoracic spine (Figure 1a), or a (2) a "tucked chin" deformity in which the angle of the jaw appears retracted (Figure 1b). The primary purposes of this study were to (1) screen lateral radiographs to determine the prevalence of these deformities in our post-instrumentation SMA type 2 population (2) use radiographic measurements to objectively characterize the deformities and (3) to set out to determine whether the sagittal deformities were present before, immediately after, or if they developed slowly over time following posterior spinal instrumentation. Additionally, we attempt to identify factors associated with deformity development. Our hypotheses were that these deformities developed slowly over time following spinal instrumentation and that a loss of thoracic kyphosis at the time of instrumentation would contribute to the deformity development.

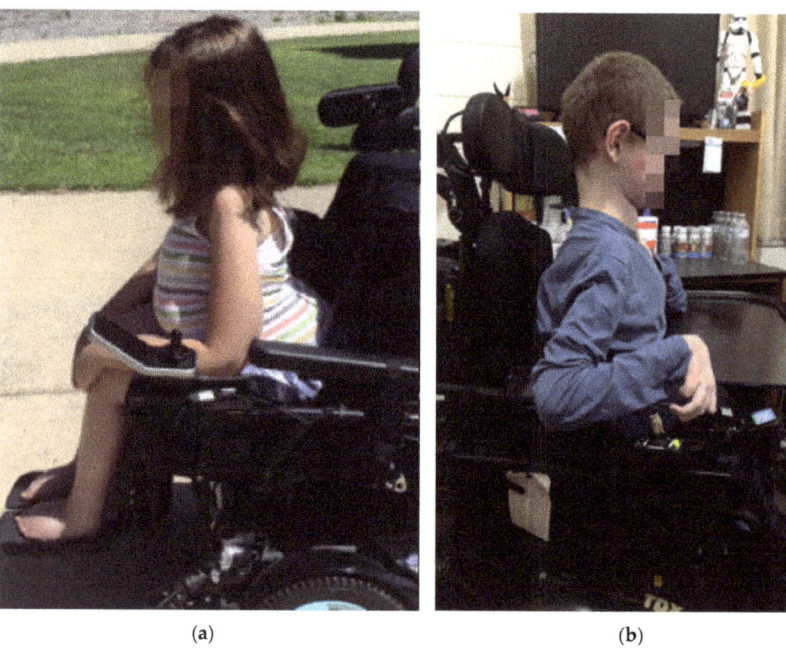

(a)　　　　　　　　　　　(b)

Figure 1. Clinical photos of "trunk tip" (**a**) and "tucked chin" (**b**) deformities. With the "trunk tip" deformity, note the space between the back of the chair and the posterior chest wall.

2. Materials and Methods

A radiographic review of SMA Type 2 patients that had undergone posterior spinal instrumentation (instrumented fusion or growing rod insertion) was performed. As we did not have standardized lateral clinical photographs of every child treated at our institution at each clinical encounter, we used the most recent lateral scoliosis radiograph as a proxy to their physical clinical examination or photographs to identify those patients who had the characteristic sagittal deformities that we have observed in either the cervical spine or trunk. The overall sagittal alignments were graded as 0 (normal), 1 (borderline), 2 (obvious) then classified as cervical ("tucked chin"), pelvic ("tipped trunk"), or both (Figure 2). Patients were then grouped into two cohorts those with or without obvious deformities (grade 0 or 1 vs. grade 2). These radiographs were reviewed and scored by a fellowship trained pediatric orthopedic spinal deformity surgeon (MAH).

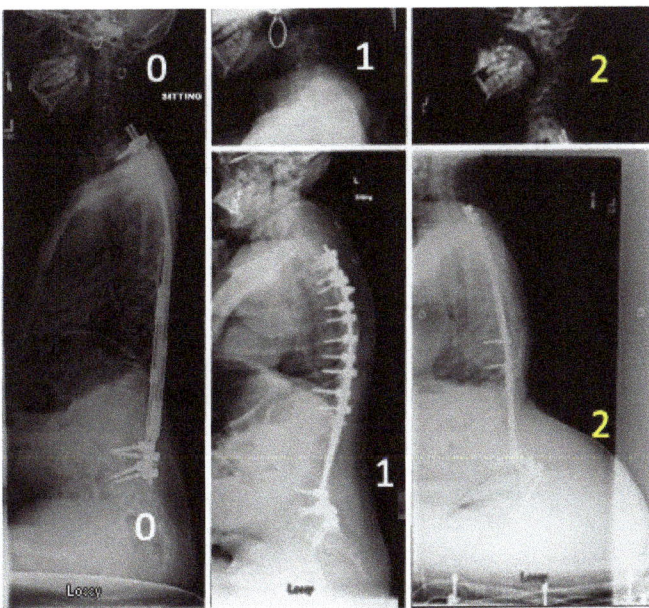

Figure 2. Examples of scoring the latest available radiographs in this study. (**Left**) Normal (0,0) scoring of no tucked chin or trunk tip. (**Middle**) Transitional scores of 1 for slight visual tucked chin (top) and prominent buttock (bottom). (**Right**) Obvious tucked chin (top) and tipped trunk (bottom) scoring a 2 in our system. Only those scoring a 2 (denoted in yellow) were included in our Deformity Cohort, these were compared against those scoring 0 or 1 (white).

Prevalence of the deformities was then determined from this data. Demographic comparisons including sex, age at surgery, and post-operative length of follow-up between cohorts was then performed. Being a tertiary referral center for these patients, some of the patients had their procedure performed at outside institutions. As such, exact operative dates were not available for every child, however the year of surgery was able to be deduced from available records. In such instances (4/32) the operative date was assigned to be December thirtieth of the operative year, to assure we were not over-estimating follow-up. To objectively characterize the deformities, "tucked chin" deformities were assessed by cervical sagittal Cobb angles and apex of deformity, while "tipped trunk" deformities were assessed by sagittal balance (C7 plumb line distance to anterior S1 endplate), Sacral Inclination (SI), and Seated Sacral Femoral Angle (SSFA) (a new measurement defined by a line tangential to the posterior sacrum and a line parallel with the anterior femoral shaft) (Figure 3). These values were then compared between those identified with and without the deformities in our screening. The same radiographic measurements described above were then performed on available pre-operative and post-operative radiographs, to assess whether these deformities were present pre-operatively, appeared in post-operative period as a result of surgery, or developed throughout the follow-up period. Finally, pelvic obliquity, coronal deformity, thoracic and lumbar sagittal Cobb angles, instrumentation levels, and hip status (reduced, subluxated, dislocated) were assessed between those with and without the obvious sagittal deformities to identify factors associated with the development of these deformities. All radiographic measurements were made using digital radiographs and measurement tools available through our clinical picture archiving and communicating system (PACS) (McKesson, San Francisco, CA, USA).

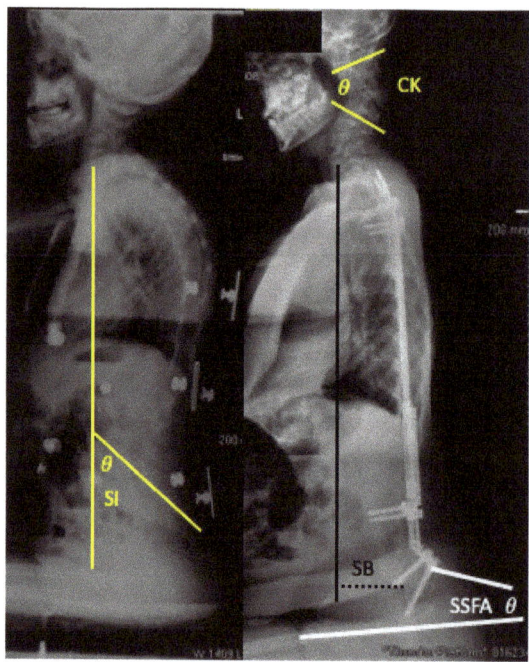

Figure 3. Examples of radiographic sagittal parameters used to objectively characterize deformities. These include Sacral Incidence (SI, Yellow); Cervical Kyphosis (CK, Yellow); Sagittal Balance (SB, Black); Seated Sacral Femoral Angle (SSFA, White).

Statistical analysis to compare the radiographic variables between those with deformity and those without was performed using an unpaired Student T-Tests. All categorical variables were assessed using Fisher's Exact test. Significance for all statistical comparisons were defined as $p < 0.05$.

3. Results

Prevalence of Obvious Deformities in our Population: Thirty-two patients with SMA type II with a history of either spinal fusion (N = 20) or growing rods (N = 12), performed between 1993 and 2015, were identified with an average of 7.6 (2.1–16.6) years post-operative follow-up. Latest lateral radiographs for each of the patients were used to grade the deformities. Obvious "tucked chin" (cervical kyphosis (N = 4)), "tipped trunk" (N = 9), or both (N = 3) deformities resulted in a total of 13/32 (40%) of the patients were identified as having a deformity, the breakdown of the scoring of the 32 can be found in Table 1. Those with deformities had significantly longer follow-up (10 (3.2–16.6) years versus 5.9 (2.1–14.7) years; $p < 0.01$) than those that did not (Table 2). No significant differences were found in the presence of the deformities between those with spinal fusion versus those with growing rods ($p = 0.76$).

Table 1. Results of screening most recent lateral radiographs for evidence of clinically recognized deformities (N = 32).

Deformity	Scoring	Tucked Chin	Trunk Tip
None	0	25	8
Mild	1	3	12
Obvious	2	4	12

Table 2. Breakdown of cohorts studied and available radiographs.

	No (Obvious) Deformity	Obvious Deformity	Prevalence
Tucked Chin	0	4	13%
Trunk Tip	0	9	28%
Any	0	13	41%
Both	0	3	9%
Follow-up Radiographs	19	13	
Upright Follow-up Radiographs	14	12	

Radiographic Characterization of Deformities: Of the 32 patients, 26 had upright follow-up radiographs available for review. As these deformities fall outside the region of instrumentation, not all measurements could be made on every film as some films were focused only on the instrumented levels (Table 3). Cervical kyphosis was greater at final follow-up (53° (37–61°) vs. −24° (−70–11°), $p < 0.001$) in those identified with a tucked chin, with the kyphotic apices in these four being located at C1-2, C2-3,C4,C5; much more proximal than classic proximal junctional kyphosis. Those identified with an obvious tipped trunk demonstrated a more positive sagittal balance (63 mm (0–165 mm) vs. 16.4 mm (−48–59 mm), $p = 0.04$) and an increased anterior tilt of the entire pelvis (demonstrated by the increased sacral inclination (SI) 74.1° (60–94°) vs. 46.8° (32–66°), $p < 0.0001$) and the decreased seated sacral femoral angle (SSFA) (2° (−13.9–8.2°) vs. 35° (8–58°), $p < 0.0001$) (Table 4).

Temporal Appearance of Deformities: The lack of standard adequate pre-operative radiographs limits interpretation of the pre-operative status of the deformities, however, no significant differences were found in mean cervical kyphosis, sagittal balance, SSFA between cohorts. Immediate post-operative radiographs also failed to demonstrate a difference between cohorts in these measurements. Post-operative SI was the only measurement found to be significantly different greater 69° (52–88°) vs. 55° (28–77°) $p = 0.03$, in those with an ultimate tucked chin or tipped trunk deformity (Table 4).

Variables Contributing to the Deformities: No differences in any of the pre-operative Cobb angles or immediate post-operative coronal or lumbosacral Cobb angles were identified over the instrumented segments between groups (Table 5).

Table 3. Demographic differences between those found with and without obvious deformities on screening.

	No Deformity	Deformity	p Value
Number of Type 2 Patients	19	13	
Age at Spinal Surgery	9.2 (4.1–19.1) years	7.9 (4.0–10.7) years	0.3
Fusion	11	9	0.71
Growing Rods	8	4	
Male:Female	7:12	6:7	0.71
Length of Clinical Post-Op Follow-up	5.9 +/− (2.1–10.5) years	10 (3.2–16.6) years	0.002
Length of Post-Op Radiographic Follow-up	5.7 (1.1–11.5) years	8.0 (1.0–16.6) years	0.1

Table 4. Sagittal parameters between those identified with and without obvious deformities on screening. Sagittal measurements were only performed on upright radiographs. These data indicate that subjective screening identified objectively measured differences. N = (number with upright lateral that allowed for each measurement/total number with upright radiographs).

Latest Follow-Up	No Deformity		Deformity		p-Value
	Average Measure	N with radiographs	Average Measure	N with radiographs	
Tucked Chin					
Cervical Sagittal Cobb (degrees)	(−)24.1 (−69.9–11.2)	(13/14)	52.5 (37.2–61.3)	(4/4 w/cervical deformity)	<0.0001
Trunk Shift					
Sagittal Balance (C7-S1) (mm)	16.4 (-48–59)	(12/14)	62.5 (0–165)	(8/12)	0.04
SI (degrees)	46.8 (32–66)	(14/14)	74.1 (60–94)	(11/12)	<0.0001
SSFA (degrees)	34.7 (7.9–57.7)	(13/14)	2.2 (−13.9–8.2)	(8/12)	<0.0001

Table 5. Temporal analysis of sagittal parameters between those that ultimately developed a deformity or did not. Lack of adequate upright radiographs limits interpretation of the data, however, from the available data no significant differences were found.

	Pre-Operative		p-Value	Immediate Post-Operative		p-Value
No Deformity (N = 19)	Average Measure	N with radiographs	No Deformity vs. Deformity	Average Measure	N with radiographs	No Deformity vs. Deformity
Cervical Sagittal Cobb	NA	0	NA	(−)10.5 (−51–28)	17	0.23
Sagittal Balance (C7-S1)	53.9 (15.3–96.4)	8	0.05	14.5 (−47.6–58.6)	19	0.43
SI	32.5 (9–56)	9	0.49	55.2 (28–77)	18	0.03
SSFA	45.5 (20.2–74.7)	8	0.88	39.6 (27–66)	17	0.16
With Deformity (N = 4/N = 13)	Average Measure	N with radiographs		Average Measure	N with radiographs	
Cervical Sagittal Cobb (N = 4)	(−)0.9 (−7.8–6.1)	2		8.5 (−57.1–44.1)	4	
Sagittal Balance (C7-S1)	7.4 (−44.3–66.7)	5		(−)2.4 (−50.7–61.4)	4	
SI	39.2 (19–56)	6		66.9 (52–88)	13	
SFA	47.8 (26.7–75.4)	5		28.8 (0–72)	13	

The lack of adequate standardized radiographs severely limits the interpretation of the preoperative data. Interestingly, the final thoracic kyphosis (throughout the instrumented levels) was significantly less in those that developed a subsequent sagittal deformity 24° (−12–46°) than in those that did not (45° (9–87°) $p = 0.008$; while lumbar lordosis was the same (Table 6). This resulted in a significantly greater overall lordotic imbalance (Defined as a sum of thoracic kyphosis-lumbar lordosis) throughout the instrumented levels in the spines that developed subsequent deformity compared to those that did not (−30° (−70°–(−)0.3°) vs. −6° (−33.9°–52.8°), $p = 0.001$). Visual inspection of residual plots produced from the linear mixed effects analysis (performed to determine statistical differences in sagittal measurements over time) failed to reveal any obvious deviations from homoscedasticity or normality and indicated a significant effect of thoracic kyphosis on the presence of deformity. Descriptive analysis did not reveal any obvious differences in the levels of instrumentation (Table 7) or in hip status (Table 8).

Table 6. Analysis of spinal parameters at each time point, comparing those with and without spinal deformities.

	Pre-Operative			Immediate Post-Operative			Latest Radiographs *			Only Upright Latest Radiographs		
	Average Measure	N^	p-Value**	Average Measure	N^	p-Value**	Average Measure	N^	p-Value**	Average Measure	N^	p-Value**
No Deformity (N = 19)												
Coronal Cobb	61.8 (30.7–118)	15*	0.65	37.2 (7.3–85.7)	19	0.14	37.5 (8.1–108)	19*	0.09	32.3 (2.7–62.6)	13	0.07
Pelvic Obliquity	28.3 (12.3–40.8)	15*	0.18	11.3 (1–56)	19	0.78	9.8 (0.4–58)	19*	0.93	9.6 (0.4–58)	13	0.97
Sagittal Cobb T/L (Kyphosis)	72.3 (41–101)	7*	0.93	37.3 (5–63)	18	0.29	44.7 (8.7–87.4)	19*	0.008	41.7 (8.7–87.4)	13	0.03
Sagittal Cobb L/S (Lordosis)	49.5 (8.3–82.2)	11*	0.92	50.6 (14–78)	19	0.36	49.2 (8.0–79.7)	17*	0.88	47.3 (8.0–79.7)	13	0.85
Kyphosis-Lordosis	26.2 (7.2–71.1)	5*	0.79	(−)16.1 (−35.6–7.4)	18	0.28	(−)5.6 (−33.9–52.8)	17*	0.001	(−)5.6 (−33.9–52.8)	13	0.005
With Deformity (N = 13)	Average Measure	N^		Average Measure	N^		Average Measure	N^		Average Measure	N^	
Coronal Cobb	56.2 (39.9–59.9)	6		27.5 (8.6–54.1)	13		21.2 (2.3–63.9)	12*		17.9 (2.3–63.9)	11	
Pelvic Obliquity	17.6 (6.5–28.5)	6		10.1 (1.2–26.4)	11		9.4 (0.2–46.5)	11		9.4 (0.2–46.5)	11	
Sagittal Cobb T/L (Kyphosis)	73.1 (51.7–94.6)	7		30.1 (−4.8–50)	11		24.2 (−11.8–46.4)	13		24.1 (−11.8–46.4)	13	
Sagittal Cobb L/S (Lordosis)	51 (16.8–77.5)	7		49.8 (37.1–76.1)	11		54.6 (37–74.2)	13		54.6 (28.6–74.2)	13	
Kyphosis-Lordosis	22.2 (−26.9–52.8)	7		(−)21 (−35.6–7.4)	10		(−)30.4 (−70.3–(−)0.3)	13		(−)30.4 (0.3–70.34)	13	

^ N = number with radiographs; * Includes supine films; ** p-value = No deformity versus deformity.

Table 7. Comparison of instrumentation between those with and without deformities.

Instrumentation		No Deformity N = 19	Deformity N = 13
Proximal	T1	2	0
	T2	12	11
	T3	3	2
	Below	2 *	0
Distal	L4 or L5	7	2
	Pelvis/Sacrum	12	11
	Revision Proximal	2 *	0
	Revision Distal	1 ^	1

* Proximal implants revised. ^ Distal implants removed and later revision.

Table 8. Comparison of hip status between those with and without deformities.

Hip Status	No Deformity N = 19	Deformity N = 13
B/L Dislocation	2	2
Unilateral Dislocation	2	0
Uni Dislocation + Uni Subluxation	5	1
B/L Subluxation	4	2
Unilateral Subluxation	3	4
B/L Reduced	0	1
Inadequate Films to Assess	3	3

4. Discussion

Scoliosis is common in all types of spinal muscular atrophy (up to 92% of patients with type 1 and 2 and 50% Type 3) and spinal deformities occur earlier with increased disease severity (Type 1 < 2 years of age, Type 2: 1–7 years of age, Type 3: 4–14 years of age) [12,13]. Posterior instrumented fusions [14–17] or distraction-based growing systems [10,11,18] have been recommended for progressive scoliotic curves in the 50–60 degree range [19]. Due to the relatively rare nature of the disease, most previous studies have grouped sub-types of SMA patients [13,16,20] or included other neuromuscular diagnoses in their analyses and reports [21–24]. These studies have focused on determining if such procedures were safe and effective [14,23] and how they affected pulmonary status [11,20,25,26], patient function and satisfaction [24,27]. While the effects of early fusion on coronal curve progression have been reported [17], no studies to date have described the effects that spinal stabilization has on the sagittal alignment above or below the instrumented levels in children with SMA.

In this study, we describe obvious deformities which occur in the sagittal plane of children with SMA type 2, above and below previously instrumented segments. For years, we have noticed these clinical deformities in our SMA population, however for the most part they have only caused seating issues, especially in those with a tipped trunk as the prominence of the buttock makes spine support difficult (Figure 1). Prior to this work, we had presumed that the children with the tipped trunk were either instrumented in excessive lordosis or perhaps there had been a gradual increase in lumbar lordosis with either continued growth or subtle loss of pelvic fixation given the known low bone density in these children [28–32]. However, after one child in our cohort required surgical treatment for severe cervical kyphosis with neurologic symptoms, we set out to critically assess how many others had such sagittal plane deformities: looking above and below the instrumented levels. In doing so, we demonstrated that these deformities are relatively common and that they are not associated with changes in lumbar lordosis (Table 6 and Figure 4).

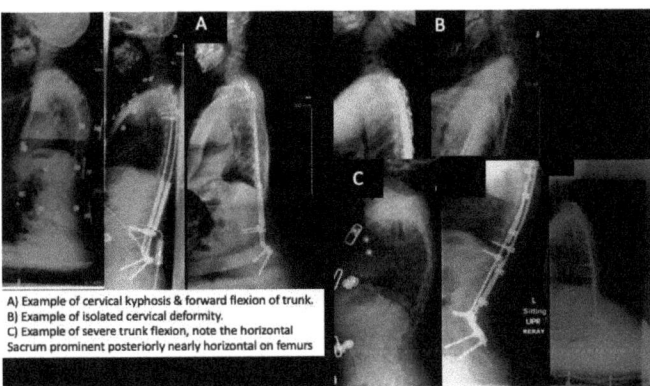

Figure 4. Examples of the cervical (**A**,**B**) and trunk deformities (**A**,**C**) developing over time.

Similar changes in sagittal alignment have been described cephalad [33–39] and/or caudal [40–42] to posterior instrumentation in children with adolescent idiopathic scoliosis. However, we are not aware of any other reports describing these changes we have observed in the SMA population. Interestingly, the opposite cervical deformity (hyperextension) has been reported following posterior spinal fusion in children with Duchenne Muscular Dystrophy [43].

From our data, it appears, that children with SMA type 2 are sensitive to hypo-kyphosis (or excessive overall relative lordosis (subtracting the lumbar lordosis from the thoracic kyphosis) following spinal instrumentation. Interestingly, little difference in kyphosis was found between cohorts immediately after surgery, but rather, that kyphosis lessened over time in those with a deformity yet increased in those without a deformity. As the cohort that developed these deformities had significantly longer follow-up, time will tell if more of these deformities develop in the remainder of these patients. As thoracic kyphosis lessened over time in the deformity group, these findings suggest that there may have been subtle anterior growth or crankshafting following the initial posterior spinal instrumentation (Figure 4). Why the average kyphosis increased over time in those without a deformity and why certain children developed cervical deformities and others trunk deformities may not be as easy to answer, as no statistical difference was found in terms of age or instrumentation type (fusion versus growing rods) (Table 3). Perhaps the increase in Sacral Incidence seen immediately post-operative contributes to the likelihood of trunk tip or that subtle preoperative cervical kyphosis or post-operative head positioning contributes to later cervical kyphosis. Lack of adequate upright pre-operative cervical imaging for every patient leaves only conjecture. The authors had hypothesized that the forward tipped trunk may occur more readily in the presence of dislocated hips as the proximal migration of the femurs may act to over lengthen the hamstrings and gluteal muscles allowing the pelvis (and the attached, fused spine) to tip forward in response to the lordotic imbalance, however our limited sample size did not support this explanation.

The lack of uniform, adequate, upright lateral radiographs is the main limitation of this study. While being a tertiary referral center for these children provided the necessary patient volume to allow recognition of the clinical deformities; it complicates assuring that all patients have uniform imaging at their referring institutions and that all images ended up in our PACS for review. This was especially true over the study period as many institutions were transitioning from standard radiographs to digital imaging during this time frame (1993–2015). Furthermore, the underlying diagnosis also complicates standard imaging as their overall weakness and spinal deformities can make upright radiographs for some impossible. Thus, while having full sets of pre-, post- and follow-up radiographs would have strengthened this study, the authors feel that the available radiographs were able to bring to light the ultimate sagittal deformities and highlights to others caring for these children the importance in obtaining AP and lateral upright sitting radiographs including the cervical spine and femurs before and after spinal surgery if possible. Furthermore, while the authors acknowledge that the lack of adequate radiographs severely limited our evaluation into the cause of the deformity, enough imaging was available to determine that at least 40% of our children with SMA type 2 and posterior instrumentation developed these deformities. As this prevalence was determined by taking those with an identified deformity and dividing that number by all the children with SMA type 2 and spinal instrumentation cared for at our institution (regardless of adequate films), additional adequate imaging would have only increased this prevalence, if more deformities had been identified.

Focusing on only SMA type 2 children may also be seen as a limitation of the current study. As children with SMA type 1 are unable to sit upright [44–46], and those with type 3 have less muscle weakness [47,48], these findings may be unique to SMA type 2 children. However, as more children are treated with the newer disease modifying drugs [49–53], the classic typing of SMA may become blurred as children become stronger [54,55]. Given the fact that the incidence of type 1 nearly doubles that of type 2 [56,57], we may find many more children with a phenotype similar to the classic SMA type 2 that may require spine surgery and develop compensatory deformities described in this study.

Exactly why these deformities develop and how best to prevent them was not completely answered in this study. It may be the result of a combination of several factors. First, the relative stiffness of the implants may result in a concentration of forces at the cephalad and caudal ends of the implants. Second, the overall muscle weakness from the disease itself results in the lack of muscular support for the unfused segments of the spine. A similar effect has been previously described as it relates to the collapse of the rib cage in children with spinal muscular atrophy known as the parasol rib deformity. [58,59] Finally, the crankshaft effect may develop with the continued growth of the anterior spinal column. Fujak et al. described the crankshaft phenomenon occurring in patients with SMA treated with telescopic rods and recommended definitive spinal fusion between the ages of 10–12 [60]. We have demonstrated safety and overall good results in these patients using standard distraction based growing rods [10,11]. While the authors would not suggest anterior spinal fusion in these children given their underlying pulmonary issues [4,20,61–63], surgical variables such as increased frequency of lengthening (using magnetically controlled devices) [64], three-column fixation (pedicle screws) [65–68] or stiffer instrumentation [69] might provide strategies to prevent the hypokyphosis from occurring. Thus, moving forward, it will be important for the spinal deformity surgeon to be aware of these potential sagittal compensations and to determine the best intervention to prevent them.

One final question that remains unanswered is the potential effect of recent disease modifying therapies on the development of the described sagittal plane deformities. The use of these therapies was not controlled for with this study as most of the study period predated the widespread use of these agents at our institution and could be the focus for future studies.

5. Conclusions

This single center, retrospective radiographic analysis demonstrated a 40% prevalence of sagittal deformities occurring above and below posterior instrumentation in SMA type 2 patients and provide radiographic parameters to assess for these deformities. While only correlative, these patients appear very sensitive to a lordotic imbalance that develops following posterior spinal instrumentation resulting in cervical kyphosis or anterior tipping (i.e., flexion) of the trunk. From this study, the authors would recommend all children with SMA being evaluated with scoliosis to have upright radiographs extending from the skull to the femurs, particularly in the lateral view, to allow for the detection of these deformities. Children with significant cervical kyphosis should be evaluated for signs of myelopathy [70], masked by their underlying neurologic pathology. The authors would also recommend caution in the complete correction or over-correction of thoracic kyphosis during spinal instrumentation. Furthermore, while only a correlative risk factor, the continued loss of thoracic kyphosis following instrumentation might be mitigated by (1) increased frequency of growing rod lengthening, (2) stiffer posterior spinal rods and (3) additional points of three-column fixation (pedicle screws), but the authors would caution against each of these interventions as they may have other unintended negative consequences. Further follow-up and studies are necessary to determine the long-term effects of these compensations and to identify strategies to avoid them.

Author Contributions: M.A.H.: Conceptualization, data curation, formal analysis, interpretation, writing—original draft preparation. R.H.: Data curation, investigation, formal analysis, writing—original draft preparation. J.B.: Formal analysis, writing—review and editing. M.T.: Data curation. S.S.: Project administration, writing—review and editing. K.P.: Writing—review and editing. K.J.N.: Resources, writing—review and editing. M.S. (Meredith Schultz): Writing—review and editing. M.K.S.: Writing—review and editing. M.S. (Mark Sharafinski): Data curation, writing—original draft preparation. B.P.H.: Writing—review and editing. All authors have read and agreed to the published version of the manuscript.

Funding: Funding was provided by UW-ICTR.

Institutional Review Board Statement: Ethical review and approval were waived for this study by the institutional Review Board at the University of Wisconsin Madison (ID number 2018-0209), due to it being secondary research for which consent was not required.

Informed Consent Statement: Not applicable.

Data Availability Statement: Data is contained within the article.

Acknowledgments: The authors would like to acknowledge support from the Cure SMA and UW-ICTR.

Conflicts of Interest: The authors declare no conflict of interest. The funders had no role in the design of the study; in the collection, analyses, or interpretation of data; in the writing of the manuscript, or in the decision to publish the results.

References

1. Munsat, T.; Davies, K. Spinal muscular atrophy 32nd ENMC International Workshop Naarden, The Netherlands, 10–12 March 1995. *Neuromuscul. Disord.* **1996**, *6*, 125–127. [CrossRef]
2. Chung, B.H.Y.; Wong, V.C.N.; Ip, P. Spinal Muscular Atrophy: Survival Pattern and Functional Status. *Pediatrics* **2004**, *114*, e548–e553. [CrossRef]
3. Durkin, E.T.; Schroth, M.K.; Helin, M.; Shaaban, A. Early laparoscopic fundoplication and gastrostomy in infants with spinal muscular atrophy type I. *J. Pediatr. Surg.* **2008**, *43*, 2031–2037. [CrossRef]
4. Finkel, R.S.; Mercuri, E.; Meyer, O.H.; Simonds, A.K.; Schroth, M.K.; Graham, R.J.; Kirschner, J.; Iannaccone, S.T.; Crawford, T.O.; Woods, S.; et al. Diagnosis and management of spinal muscular atrophy: Part 2: Pulmonary and acute care; medications, supplements and immunizations; other organ systems; and ethics. *Neuromuscul. Disord.* **2018**, *28*, 197–207. [CrossRef]
5. Halanski, M.A.; Patterson, K.G.; Sund, S.A.; Makholm, L.M.; Schroth, M.K. Assessing the Needs of the SMA Population. Survey Results of Healthcare Providers and Families. *Sage Open* **2014**, *4*, 1–5. [CrossRef]
6. Kissel, J.T.; Scott, C.B.; Reyna, S.P.; Crawford, T.O.; Simard, L.R.; Krosschell, K.J.; Acsadi, G.; Elsheik, B.; Schroth, M.K.; D'Anjou, G.; et al. SMA CARNI-VAL TRIAL PART II: A Prospective, Single-Armed Trial of L-Carnitine and Valproic Acid in Ambulatory Children with Spinal Muscular Atrophy. *PLoS ONE* **2011**, *6*, e21296. [CrossRef] [PubMed]
7. Krosschell, K.J.; Kissel, J.T.; Townsend, E.L.; Simeone, S.D.; Zhang, R.Z.; Reyna, S.P.; Crawford, T.O.; Schroth, M.K.; Acsadi, G.; Kishnani, P.S.; et al. Clinical trial of L-Carnitine and valproic acid in spinal muscular atrophy type I. *Muscle Nerve* **2018**, *57*, 193–199. [CrossRef] [PubMed]
8. Mercuri, E.; Finkel, R.S.; Muntoni, F.; Wirth, B.; Montes, J.; Main, M.; Mazzone, E.S.; Vitale, M.; Snyder, B.; Quijano-Roy, S.; et al. Diagnosis and management of spinal muscular atrophy: Part 1: Recommendations for diagnosis, rehabilitation, orthopedic and nutritional care. *Neuromuscul. Disord.* **2018**, *28*, 103–115. [CrossRef] [PubMed]

9. Wang, C.H.; Finkel, R.S.; Bertini, E.; Schroth, M.; Simonds, A.; Wong, B.; Aloysius, A.; Morrison, L.; Main, M.; Crawford, T.O.; et al. Consensus Statement for Standard of Care in Spinal Muscular Atrophy. *J. Child Neurol.* **2007**, *22*, 1027–1049. [CrossRef]
10. Chandran, S.; McCarthy, J.; Noonan, K.; Mann, D.; Nemeth, B.; Guiliani, T. Early Treatment of Scoliosis with Growing Rods in Children with Severe Spinal Muscular atrophy: A preliminary report. *J. Pediatr. Orthop.* **2011**, *31*, 450–454. [CrossRef]
11. Lenhart, R.L.; Youlo, S.; Schroth, M.K.; Noonan, K.J.; McCarthy, J.; Mann, D.; Hetzel, S.; Sund, S.A.; Halanski, M.A. Radiographic and Respiratory Effects of Growing Rods in Children with Spinal Muscular Atrophy. *J. Pediatr. Orthop.* **2017**, *37*, e500–e504. [CrossRef]
12. Evans, G.A.; Drennan, J.C.; Russman, B.S. Functional classification and orthopaedic management of spinal muscular atrophy. *J. Bone Joint Surg. Br.* **1981**, *63B*, 516–522. [CrossRef]
13. Fujak, A.; Raab, W.; Schuh, A.; Richter, S.; Forst, R.; Forst, J. Natural course of scoliosis in proximal spinal muscular atrophy type II and IIIa: Descriptive clinical study with retrospective data collection of 126 patients. *BMC Musculoskelet. Disord.* **2013**, *14*, 283. [CrossRef]
14. Granata, C.; Cervellati, S.; Ballestrazzi, A.; Corbascio, M.; Merlini, L. Spine surgery in spinal muscular atrophy: Long-term results. *Neuromuscul. Disord.* **1993**, *3*, 207–215. [CrossRef]
15. Merlini, L.; Granata, C.; Bonfiglioli, S.; Marini, M.L.; Cervellati, S.; Savini, R. Scoliosis in spinal muscular atrophy: Natural history and management. *Dev. Med. Child Neurol.* **1989**, *31*, 501–508. [CrossRef] [PubMed]
16. Rodillo, E.; Marini, M.; Heckmatt, J.; Dubowitz, V. Scoliosis in Spinal Muscular Atrophy: Review of 63 Cases. *J. Child Neurol.* **1989**, *4*, 118–123. [CrossRef] [PubMed]
17. Zebala, L.P.; Bridwell, K.H.; Baldus, C.; Richards, S.B.; Dormans, J.P.; Lenke, L.G.; Auerbach, J.D.; Lovejoy, J. Minimum 5-year Radiographic Results of Long Scoliosis Fusion in Juvenile Spinal Muscular Atrophy patients: Major curve progression after instrumented fusion. *J. Pediatr. Orthop.* **2011**, *31*, 480–488. [CrossRef] [PubMed]
18. McElroy, M.J.; Shaner, A.C.; Crawford, T.O.; Thompson, G.H.; Kadakia, R.V.; Akbarnia, B.A.; Skaggs, D.L.; Emans, J.B.; Sponseller, P.D. Growing rods for scoliosis in spinal muscular atrophy: Structural effects, complications, and hospital stays. *Spine* **2011**, *36*, 1305–1311. [CrossRef] [PubMed]
19. Sucato, D.J. Spine Deformity in Spinal Muscular Atrophy. *J. Bone Jt. Surgery Am. Vol.* **2007**, *89*, 148–154. (In English) [CrossRef]
20. Chng, S.Y.; Wong, Y.Q.; Hui, J.H.; Wong, H.K.; Ong, H.T.; Goh, D.Y. Pulmonary function and scoliosis in children with spinal muscular atrophy types II and III. *J. Paediatr. Child Health* **2003**, *39*, 673–676. [CrossRef]
21. Bentley, G.; Haddad, F.; Bull, T.M.; Seingry, D. The treatment of scoliosis in muscular dystrophy using modified Luque and Harrington-Luque instrumentation. *J. Bone Jt. Surgery. Br. Vol.* **2001**, *83*, 22–28. [CrossRef]
22. Modi, H.; Suh, S.-W.; Hong, J.-Y.; Cho, J.-W.; Park, J.-H.; Yang, J.-H. Treatment and complications in flaccid neuromuscular scoliosis (Duchenne muscular dystrophy and spinal muscular atrophy) with posterior-only pedicle screw instrumentation. *Eur. Spine J.* **2009**, *19*, 384–393. [CrossRef] [PubMed]
23. Modi, H.; Suh, S.-W.; Hong, J.-Y.; Park, Y.-H.; Yang, J.-H. Surgical Correction of Paralytic Neuromuscular Scoliosis with Poor Pulmonary Functions. *J. Spinal Disord. Tech.* **2011**, *24*, 325–333. [CrossRef]
24. Bridwell, K.H.; Baldus, C.; Iffrig, T.M.; Lenke, L.G.; Blanke, K. Process Measures and Patient/Parent Evaluation of Surgical Management of Spinal Deformities in Patients with Progressive Flaccid Neuromuscular Scoliosis (Duchenne's Muscular Dystrophy and Spinal Muscular Atrophy). *Spine* **1999**, *24*, 1300–1309. [CrossRef] [PubMed]
25. Robinson, D.; Galasko, C.S.; Delaney, C.; Williamson, J.B.; Barrie, J.L. Scoliosis and lung function in spinal muscular atrophy. *Eur. Spine J.* **1995**, *4*, 268–273. [CrossRef]
26. Chong, H.S.; Moon, E.S.; Kim, H.S.; Ankur, N.; Park, J.O.; Kim, J.Y.; Kho, P.A.B.; Moon, S.H.; Lee, H.M.; Seul, N.H. Comparison between Operated Muscular Dystrophy and Spinal Muscular Atrophy Patients in terms of Radiological, Pulmonary and Functional Outcomes. *Asian Spine J.* **2010**, *4*, 82–88. [CrossRef]
27. Aprin, H.; Bowen, J.R.; MacEwen, G.D.; Hall, J.E. Spine fusion in patients with spinal muscular atrophy. *J. Bone Jt. Surgery Am. Vol.* **1982**, *64*, 1179–1187. [CrossRef]
28. Khatri, I.A.; Chaudhry, U.S.; Seikaly, M.G.; Browne, R.H.; Iannaccone, S.T. Low Bone Mineral Density in Spinal Muscular Atrophy. *J. Clin. Neuromuscul. Dis.* **2008**, *10*, 11–17. [CrossRef]
29. Lee, B.J.; Cox, G.A.; Maddatu, T.P.; Judex, S.; Rubin, C.T. Devastation of bone tissue in the appendicular skeleton parallels the progression of neuromuscular disease. *J. Musculoskelet. Neuronal Interact.* **2009**, *9*, 215–224.
30. Shanmugarajan, S.; Swoboda, K.; Iannaccone, S.T.; Ries, W.L.; Maria, B.L.; Reddy, S.V. Congenital Bone Fractures in Spinal Muscular Atrophy: Functional Role for SMN Protein in Bone Remodeling. *J. Child Neurol.* **2007**, *22*, 967–973. [CrossRef] [PubMed]
31. Shanmugarajan, S.; Tsuruga, E.; Swoboda, K.; Maria, B.L.; Ries, W.L.; Reddy, S.V. Bone loss in survival motor neuron (Smn −/− SMN2) genetic mouse model of spinal muscular atrophy. *J. Pathol.* **2009**, *219*, 52–60. [CrossRef] [PubMed]
32. Wasserman, H.M.; Hornung, L.N.; Stenger, P.J.; Rutter, M.M.; Wong, B.L.; Rybalsky, I.; Khoury, J.C.; Kalkwarf, H.J. Low bone mineral density and fractures are highly prevalent in pediatric patients with spinal muscular atrophy regardless of disease severity. *Neuromuscul. Disord.* **2017**, *27*, 331–337. [CrossRef] [PubMed]
33. Tauchi, R.; Kawakami, N.; Ohara, T.; Saito, T.; Tanabe, H.; Morishita, K.; Yamauchi, I. Sagittal Alignment Profile Following Selective Thoracolumbar/Lumbar Fusion in Patients with Lenke Type 5C Adolescent Idiopathic Scoliosis. *Spine* **2019**, *44*, 1193–1200. [CrossRef] [PubMed]

34. Berger, R.J.; Sultan, A.A.; Tanenbaum, J.E.; Cantrell, W.A.; Gurd, D.P.; Kuivila, T.E.; Mroz, T.E.; Steinmetz, M.P.; Goodwin, R.C. Cervical sagittal alignment and the impact of posterior spinal instrumented fusion in patients with Lenke type 1 adolescent idiopathic scoliosis. *J. Spine Surg.* **2018**, *4*, 342–348. [CrossRef]
35. Zhao, J.; Chen, Z.; Yang, M.; Li, G.; Zhao, Y.; Li, M. Does spinal fusion to T2, T3, or T4 affects sagittal alignment of the cervical spine in Lenke 1 AIS: A retrospective study. *Medicine* **2018**, *97*, e9764. [CrossRef]
36. Zhang, Z.; Liu, Z.; Zhu, Z.; Qiu, Y. Predictors of ultimate postoperative cervical sagittal alignment in main thoracic adolescent idiopathic scoliosis: A long-term follow-up study. *Medicine* **2017**, *96*, e8799. [CrossRef]
37. Cho, J.H.; Hwang, C.J.; Choi, Y.H.; Lee, D.-H.; Lee, C.S. Cervical sagittal alignment in patients with adolescent idiopathic scoliosis: Is it corrected by surgery? *J. Neurosurg. Pediatr.* **2018**, *21*, 292–301. [CrossRef]
38. Hayashi, K.; Toyoda, H.; Terai, H.; Suzuki, A.; Hoshino, M.; Tamai, K.; Ohyama, S.; Nakamura, H. Cervical lordotic alignment following posterior spinal fusion for adolescent idiopathic scoliosis: Reciprocal changes and risk factors for malalignment. *J. Neurosurg. Pediatr.* **2017**, *19*, 440–447. [CrossRef]
39. Canavese, F.; Sussman, M.D. Strategies of hip management in neuromuscular disorders: Duchenne Muscular Dystrophy, Spinal Muscular Atrophy, Charcot-Marie-Tooth Disease and Arthrogryposis Multiplex Congenita. *Hip Int.* **2009**, *19* (Suppl. 6), S46–S52. [CrossRef]
40. Dumpa, S.R.; Shetty, A.P.; Aiyer, S.N.; Kanna, R.M.; Rajasekaran, S. Reciprocal Changes in Sagittal Alignment in Adolescent Idiopathic Scoliosis Patients Following Strategic Pedicle Screw Fixation. *Asian Spine J.* **2018**, *12*, 300–308. [CrossRef]
41. Day, L.M.; Ramchandran, S.; Jalai, C.M.; Diebo, B.G.; Liabaud, B.; Lafage, R.; Protopsaltis, T.; Passias, P.G.; Schwab, F.J.; Bess, S.; et al. Thoracolumbar Realignment Surgery Results in Simultaneous Reciprocal Changes in Lower Extremities and Cervical Spine. *Spine* **2017**, *42*, 799–807. [CrossRef]
42. Matsumoto, H.; Colacchio, N.D.; Schwab, F.J.; Lafage, V.; Roye, D.P.; Vitale, M.G. Flatback Revisited: Reciprocal Loss of Lumbar Lordosis Following Selective Thoracic Fusion in the Setting of Adolescent Idiopathic Scoliosis. *Spine Deform.* **2015**, *3*, 345–351. [CrossRef] [PubMed]
43. Granata, C.; Merlini, L.; Cervellati, S.; Ballestrazzi, A.; Giannini, S.; Corbascio, M.; Lari, S. Long-term results of spine surgery in Duchenne muscular dystrophy. *Neuromuscul. Disord.* **1996**, *6*, 61–68. [CrossRef]
44. Oskoui, M.; Levy, G.; Garland, C.J.; Gray, J.M.; O'Hagen, J.; De Vivo, D.C.; Kaufmann, P. The changing natural history of spinal muscular atrophy type 1. *Neurology* **2007**, *69*, 1931–1936. [CrossRef] [PubMed]
45. Bertini, E.; Mercuri, E. A prospective natural history study of type 1 spinal muscular atrophy. *Nat. Rev. Neurol.* **2018**, *14*, 197–198. [CrossRef] [PubMed]
46. Kolb, S.J.; Coffey, C.S.; Yankey, J.W.; Pt, D.K.K.; Arnold, W.D.; Rutkove, S.; Swoboda, K.; Reyna, S.P.; Sakonju, A.; Darras, B.; et al. Natural history of infantile-onset spinal muscular atrophy. *Ann. Neurol.* **2017**, *82*, 883–891. [CrossRef] [PubMed]
47. Kaufmann, P.; McDermott, M.P.; Darras, B.T.; Finkel, R.; Kang, P.; Oskoui, M.; Constantinescu, A.; Sproule, D.M.; Foley, A.R.; Yang, M.; et al. Observational study of spinal muscular atrophy type 2 and 3: Functional outcomes over 1 year. *Arch. Neurol.* **2011**, *68*, 779–786. [CrossRef] [PubMed]
48. Wirth, B.; Brichta, L.; Schrank, B.; Lochmüller, H.; Blick, S.; Baasner, A.; Heller, R. Mildly affected patients with spinal muscular atrophy are partially protected by an increased SMN2 copy number. *Hum. Genet.* **2006**, *119*, 422–428. [CrossRef]
49. Mendell, J.R.; Al-Zaidy, S.; Shell, R.; Arnold, W.D.; Rodino-Klapac, L.R.; Prior, T.W.; Lowes, L.; Alfano, L.; Berry, K.; Church, K.; et al. Single-Dose Gene-Replacement Therapy for Spinal Muscular Atrophy. *N. Engl. J. Med.* **2017**, *377*, 1713–1722. [CrossRef]
50. Mercuri, E.; Darras, B.; Chiriboga, C.A.; Day, J.W.; Campbell, C.; Connolly, A.M.; Iannaccone, S.T.; Kirschner, J.; Kuntz, N.L.; Saito, K.; et al. Nusinersen versus Sham Control in Later-Onset Spinal Muscular Atrophy. *N. Engl. J. Med.* **2018**, *378*, 625–635. [CrossRef]
51. Paton, D. Nusinersen: Antisense oligonucleotide to increase SMN protein production in spinal muscular atrophy. *Drugs Today* **2017**, *53*, 327–337. [CrossRef]
52. Finkel, R.S.; Chiriboga, C.A.; Vajsar, J.; Day, J.W.; Montes, J.; De Vivo, D.C.; Yamashita, M.; Rigo, F.; Hung, G.; Schneider, E.; et al. Treatment of infantile-onset spinal muscular atrophy with nusinersen: A phase 2, open-label, dose-escalation study. *Lancet* **2016**, *388*, 3017–3026. [CrossRef]
53. Farrar, M.A.; Park, S.B.; Vucic, S.; Carey, K.; Turner, B.; Gillingwater, T.; Swoboda, K.; Kiernan, M.C. Emerging therapies and challenges in spinal muscular atrophy. *Ann. Neurol.* **2017**, *81*, 355–368. [CrossRef] [PubMed]
54. Tizzano, E.F.; Finkel, R.S. Spinal muscular atrophy: A changing phenotype beyond the clinical trials. *Neuromuscul. Disord.* **2017**, *27*, 883–889. [CrossRef] [PubMed]
55. Finkel, R.S.; Mercuri, E.; Darras, B.; Connolly, A.M.; Kuntz, N.L.; Kirschner, J.; Chiriboga, C.A.; Saito, K.; Servais, L.; Tizzano, E.; et al. Nusinersen versus Sham Control in Infantile-Onset Spinal Muscular Atrophy. *N. Engl. J. Med.* **2017**, *377*, 1723–1732. [CrossRef] [PubMed]
56. Ogino, S.; Wilson, R.B. Spinal muscular atrophy: Molecular genetics and diagnostics. *Expert Rev. Mol. Diagn.* **2004**, *4*, 15–29. [CrossRef]
57. Verhaart, I.E.C.; Robertson, A.; Wilson, I.J.; Aartsma-Rus, A.; Cameron, S.; Jones, C.C.; Cook, S.F.; Lochmüller, H. Prevalence, incidence and carrier frequency of 5q–linked spinal muscular atrophy—A literature review. *Orphanet J. Rare Dis.* **2017**, *12*, 1–15. [CrossRef]
58. Schwentker, E.P.; Gibson, D.A. The orthopaedic aspects of spinal muscular atrophy. *J. Bone Jt. Surgery Am. Vol.* **1976**, *58*, 32–38. [CrossRef]

59. Schroth, M.K. Special Considerations in the Respiratory Management of Spinal Muscular Atrophy: FIGURE 1. *Pediatrics* **2009**, *123*, S245–S249. [CrossRef] [PubMed]
60. Fujak, A.; Raab, W.; Schuh, A.; Kreß, A.; Forst, R.; Forst, J. Operative treatment of scoliosis in proximal spinal muscular atrophy: Results of 41 patients. *Arch. Orthop. Trauma Surg.* **2012**, *132*, 1697–1706. [CrossRef] [PubMed]
61. Holt, J.; Dolan, L.A.; Weinstein, S.L. Outcomes of Primary Posterior Spinal Fusion for Scoliosis in Spinal Muscular Atrophy: Clinical, Radiographic, and Pulmonary Outcomes and Complications. *J. Pediatr. Orthop.* **2017**, *37*, e505–e511. [CrossRef]
62. Chou, S.-H.; Lin, G.-T.; Shen, P.-C.; Lue, Y.-J.; Lu, C.-C.; Tien, Y.-C.; Lu, Y.-M. The effect of scoliosis surgery on pulmonary function in spinal muscular atrophy type II patients. *Eur. Spine J.* **2017**, *26*, 1721–1731. [CrossRef]
63. Chua, K.; Tan, C.Y.; Chen, Z.; Wong, H.K.; Lee, E.H.; Tay, S.K.; Ong, H.T.; Goh, D.Y.; Hui, J.H. Long-term Follow-up of Pulmonary Function and Scoliosis in Patients with Duchenne's Muscular Dystrophy and Spinal Muscular Atrophy. *J. Pediatr. Orthop.* **2016**, *36*, 63–69. [CrossRef] [PubMed]
64. Lorenz, H.M.; Badwan, B.; Hecker, M.M.; Tsaknakis, K.; Groenefeld, K.; Braunschweig, L.; Hell, A.K. Magnetically Controlled Devices Parallel to the Spine in Children with Spinal Muscular Atrophy. *JBJS Open Access* **2017**, *2*, e0036. [CrossRef]
65. Murphy, R.F.; Mooney, J.F. The Crankshaft Phenomenon. *J. Am. Acad. Orthop. Surg.* **2017**, *25*, e185–e193. [CrossRef]
66. Tao, F.; Zhao, Y.; Wu, Y.; Xie, Y.; Li, M.; Lu, Y.; Pan, F.; Guo, F.; Li, F. The Effect of Differing Spinal Fusion Instrumentation on the Occurrence of Postoperative Crankshaft Phenomenon in Adolescent Idiopathic Scoliosis. *J. Spinal Disord. Tech.* **2010**, *23*, e75–e80. [CrossRef] [PubMed]
67. Şarlak, A.Y.; Atmaca, H.; Tosun, B.; Musaoğlu, R.; Buluç, L. Isolated Pedicle Screw Instrumented Correction for the Treatment of Thoracic Congenital Scoliosis. *J. Spinal Disord. Tech.* **2010**, *23*, 525–529. [CrossRef]
68. Kioschos, H.C.; Asher, M.A.; Lark, R.G.; Harner, E.J. Overpowering the Crankshaft mechanism. The effect of posterior spinal fusion with and without stiff transpedicular fixation on anterior spinal column growth in immature canines. *Spine* **1996**, *21*, 1168–1173. [CrossRef]
69. Burton, D.C.; Asher, M.A.; Lai, S.M. Scoliosis Correction Maintenance in Skeletally Immature Patients with Idiopathic scoliosis. Is anterior fusion really necessary? *Spine* **2000**, *25*, 61–68. [CrossRef] [PubMed]
70. Bernatz, J.T.; Anderson, P.A.; Halanski, M.A. Cervical Kyphosis in Spinal Muscular Atrophy: A Case Report. *JBJS Case Connect.* **2020**, *10*, e19. [CrossRef]

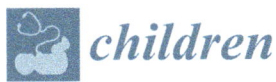 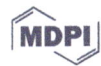

Case Report

Expanding the Phenotypic Spectrum of *ECEL1*-Associated Distal Arthrogryposis

Akshata Huddar [1], Kiran Polavarapu [2], Veeramani Preethish-Kumar [1], Mainak Bardhan [1], Gopikrishnan Unnikrishnan [1], Saraswati Nashi [1], Seena Vengalil [1], Priyanka Priyadarshini [3], Karthik Kulanthaivelu [3], Gautham Arunachal [4], Hanns Lochmüller [2] and Atchayaram Nalini [1,*]

1 Department of Neurology, National Institute of Mental Health and Neuro-Sciences, Bengaluru 560029, India; akshatahuddar@yahoo.com (A.H.); prthshkumar@gmail.com (V.P.-K.); bardhan.mainak@gmail.com (M.B.); gopikrishnanu@gmail.com (G.U.); nandanashi@gmail.com (S.N.); seenavengalil@gmail.com (S.V.)
2 Children's Hospital of Eastern Ontario Research Institute, Department of Medicine, Division of Neurology, The Ottawa Hospital, Brain and Mind Research Institute, University of Ottawa, Ottawa, ON K1H 8L1, Canada; kpolavarapu@cheo.on.ca (K.P.); hlochmuller@toh.ca (H.L.)
3 Department of Neuro Imaging and Interventional Radiology, National Institute of Mental Health and Neuro-Sciences, Bengaluru 560029, India; priyankapriyadarshini1986@gmail.com (P.P.); pammalkk@gmail.com (K.K.)
4 Department of Human Genetics, National Institute of Mental Health and Neuro-Sciences, Bengaluru 560029, India; gautham.arunachal@gmail.com
* Correspondence: atchayaramnalini@yahoo.co.in; Tel.: +91-80-26995139; Fax: +91-80-26564830

Citation: Huddar, A.; Polavarapu, K.; Preethish-Kumar, V.; Bardhan, M.; Unnikrishnan, G.; Nashi, S.; Vengalil, S.; Priyadarshini, P.; Kulanthaivelu, K.; Arunachal, G.; et al. Expanding the Phenotypic Spectrum of *ECEL1*-Associated Distal Arthrogryposis. *Children* 2021, 8, 909. https://doi.org/10.3390/children8100909

Academic Editor: Rudolf Korinthenberg

Received: 30 July 2021
Accepted: 6 October 2021
Published: 13 October 2021

Publisher's Note: MDPI stays neutral with regard to jurisdictional claims in published maps and institutional affiliations.

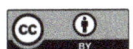

Copyright: © 2021 by the authors. Licensee MDPI, Basel, Switzerland. This article is an open access article distributed under the terms and conditions of the Creative Commons Attribution (CC BY) license (https://creativecommons.org/licenses/by/4.0/).

Abstract: Distal arthrogryposis type 5D (DA5D), a rare autosomal recessive disorder, is caused by mutations in *ECEL1*. We describe two consanguineous families (three patients) with novel *ECEL1* gene mutations detected by next-generation sequencing (NGS). A 12-year-old boy (patient 1) presented with birth asphyxia, motor developmental delay, multiple joint contractures, pes planus, kyphoscoliosis, undescended testis, hypophonic speech with a nasal twang, asymmetric ptosis, facial weakness, absent abductor pollicis brevis, bifacial, and distal lower limb weakness. Muscle MRI revealed asymmetric fatty infiltration of tensor fascia lata, hamstring, lateral compartment of the leg, and gastrocnemius. In addition, 17-year-old monozygotic twins (patients 2 and 3) presented with motor development delay, white hairlock, hypertelorism, tented upper lip, bulbous nose, tongue furrowing, small low set ears, multiple contractures, pes cavus, prominent hyperextensibility at the knee, hypotonia of lower limbs, wasting and weakness of all limbs (distal > proximal), areflexia, and high steppage gait. One had perinatal insult, seizures, mild intellectual disability, unconjugated eye movements, and primary optic atrophy. In the twins, MRI revealed extensive fatty infiltration of the gluteus maximus, quadriceps, hamstrings, and anterior and posterior compartment of the leg. Electrophysiology showed prominent motor axonopathy. NGS revealed rare homozygous missense variants c.602T > C (p.Met201Thr) in patient 1 and c.83C > T (p.Ala28Val) in patients 2 and 3, both localized in exon 2 of *ECEL1* gene. Our three cases expand the clinical, imaging, and molecular spectrum of the *ECEL1*-mutation-related DA5D.

Keywords: distal arthrogryposis; AMC; *ECEL1*; contractures; muscle MRI

1. Introduction

Arthrogryposis multiplex congenita (AMC) is a heterogeneous group of disorders characterized by multiple nonprogressive congenital joint contractures involving at least two different body parts [1]. Distal arthrogryposis (DAs) is diagnosed when contractures mainly involve distal joints of hands, feet, wrist, and ankle [1,2]. DAs are caused by mutations in genes encoding contractile proteins of skeletal myofibers and are further subdivided into 10 different phenotypic and genetic forms caused by *TPM2*, *TNNI2*, *TNNT3*, *MYH3*, *MYBPC1*, *MYH8*, *FBN2*, *PIEZO2*, and *ECEL1* [2,3]. Distal arthrogryposis type 5D (DA5D; OMIM 108145) is described as a rare autosomal recessive DA unlike other dominant forms and has a wide phenotypic spectrum including joint contractures, camptodactyly, hip dislocation, scoliosis, lower limb atrophy, clubfoot, dysmorphic features, furrowed tongue, and asymmetric or unilateral ptosis. Typically, there is normal intelligence and an absence of ophthalmoplegia [3,4]. DA5D is caused due to compound heterozygous or homozygous mutations in membrane-bound metalloprotease endothelin-converting enzyme-like 1 (*ECEL1* (OMIM 605896), also termed DINE in rodents) [3,5]. *ECEL1* is predominantly expressed in neuronal cells and plays an important role in the final axonal arborization of motor nerves to the endplate of skeletal muscles, resulting in the poor formation of the neuromuscular junction [3,5]. We describe two families with three affected individuals with novel *ECEL1* gene mutations with additional features, which thus expands the clinical and imaging spectrum of DA5D.

2. Materials and Methods

2.1. Patients

The patients were identified and thoroughly investigated with standard clinical and electrophysiological examinations at the specialized neurology and neuromuscular clinic, Department of Neurology, National Institute of Mental Health and Neurosciences, India. Institutional Ethics committee approval (NIMHANS/IEC/2020-21) was obtained to collect all clinical, electrophysiological, and genetic data from the medical records. Patients and parents provided written informed consent to publish the patient's details, along with face recognition in the clinical photographs and videos. All evaluated patients underwent a thorough clinical examination, and details were recorded in a pre-designed proforma.

2.2. Genetic Analysis

The DNA was extracted from blood samples using the QIAamp DNA Blood Mini Kit (QIAGEN, Hilden, Germany). We analyzed both families by Trios next-generation sequencing (NGS) for identification of a genetic cause. Patient 1, along with parents in family 1, underwent whole-exome sequencing (exome research panel by integrated DNA technologies (Coralville, IA, USA) having 39 mb probe span of the human genome and covering coding regions of 19,396 genes) with a mean sequencing coverage of >50–60 X on Illumina (San Diego, CA, USA) sequencing platform. Patients 2 and 3, along with parents in family 2, underwent clinical exome sequencing (custom panel by Agilent technologies (Santa Clara, CA, USA) having 29 mb probe span covering coding regions of 8332 known disease-associated genes) with a mean sequencing coverage of >80–100 X on Illumina sequencing platform. Bioinformatic analysis was concentrated on the analysis of significant variants in 48 known hereditary arthrogryposes and congenital myasthenic syndrome genes for patient 1 and 123 known genes associated with hereditary neuropathies and arthrogryposis/congenital myasthenic syndromes for patients 2 and 3 (Tables S1 and S2). Germ-line variants were identified by aligning the obtained sequences to the human reference genome (GRCh37/hg19) using the BWA program and analyzed using the Genome Analysis Toolkit best-practices variant-calling pipeline [6,7]. The variants were annotated using the Ensemble (release 89) human gene model, with disease annotations ClinVar, SwissVar, and the licensed Human Gene Mutation Database; population frequencies from the 1000 Genome Phase 3, ExAC, gnomAD, and dbSNP databases, and the internal Indian-specific database, as well as in silico prediction algorithms in PolyPhen-2, SIFT, Mutation Taster 2, and LRT. The pathogenicity of the variants was assessed based on 2015 American College of Medical Genetics (ACMG) guidelines [8].

3. Results

Family 1: patient 1 was a 12-year-old boy evaluated in the year 2016. He was born to consanguineous parents at term by forceps delivery following an uneventful antenatal period and birth weight of 2.25 kg. There was a history of birth asphyxia (delayed cry at birth and neonatal intensive care unit (NICU) stay for one week). He had foot deformities (pes planus, right eqinovarus) at birth. There was a motor developmental delay, normal mental functions, progressive ptosis, limitation of movement at elbow and hip, and altered gait. He had phimosis, undescended testis, and recurrent urinary tract infection. On examination, he had long eyelashes, low set ears, trismus, high arched palate, asymmetrical ptosis, left eye proptosis with normal fundus, complete extraocular muscle movements, bifacial weakness, hypophonic speech with a nasal twang, taut skin of fingers and face, ulnar deviation of the wrist, absent abductor pollicis brevis, severe contractures of fingers with flexion deformity, contractures at elbows, hip, knee and ankle, pes planus, right side equinovarus deformity, kyphoscoliosis, and calf atrophy with mild distal limb weakness (Medical Research Council grade (MRC) 4) and preserved tendon reflexes (Figure 1).

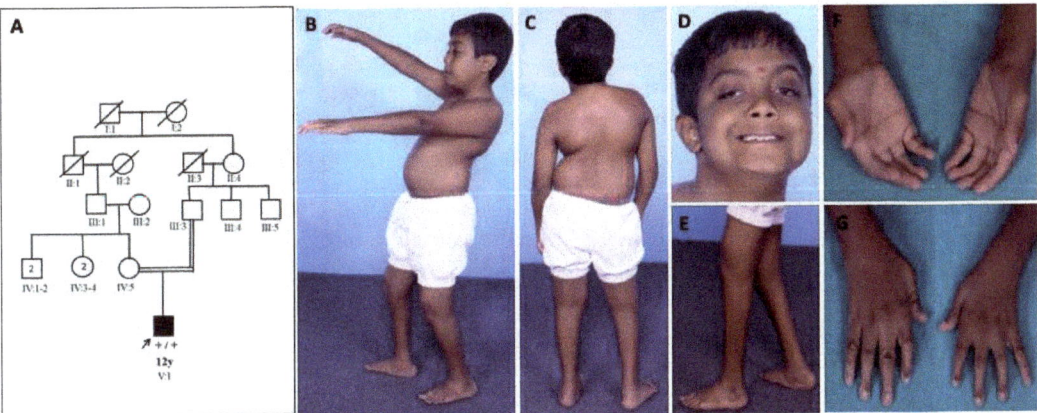

Figure 1. Pedigree and clinical images of patient 1 with DA5D: (**A**) pedigree of family 1; (**B,C**) kyphoscoliosis with bilateral hip and knee contracture; (**D**) asymmetric ptosis; (**E**) calf atrophy, contracture at the knee, pes planus, prominent calcaneum; (**F,G**) contractures of fingers with absent abductor pollicis brevis.

He was able to walk independently with a limp and mild waddling. Diagnosis of arthrogryposis multiplex congenita (AMC) was considered. Muscle MRI revealed asymmetric fatty infiltration (right > left) in tensor fascia lata, hamstring, lateral compartment of the right leg, and gastrocnemius (Figure 2). Brain MRI was normal. At the last follow-up (17 years of age) during July 2021, the clinical condition was stationary.

Family 2: patient 2 was a 17-year-old-boy evaluated during June 2018. He is the first of the twins, born to consanguineous parents at term by normal vaginal delivery following an uneventful antenatal period, and had a birth weight of 1.75 kg (<5th percentile). Fetal movements were normal. He did not cry at birth and had recurrent seizures from day 3 of life and was kept in NICU for 1 week. Subsequently, the child was noticed to have delayed acquisition of all milestones, mild intellectual disability, and recurrent seizures since 8 years of age. He has never been able to walk independently, has altered high stepping gait with slowly progressive weakness of all limbs. Examination revealed flat occiput, hypertelorism, tented upper lip, bushy eyebrows, small low set ears, bulbous nose, a central deep furrow of the tongue, white hairlock, unconjugated eye movements, nonparalytic squint, primary optic atrophy, normal extraocular movements, bifacial weakness, small hands and fingers, asymmetric contractures at fingers (metacarpophalangeal and interphalangeal joints), wrist in extension, and elbow with prominent hyperextensibility at the knees and pes cavus (Figure 3).

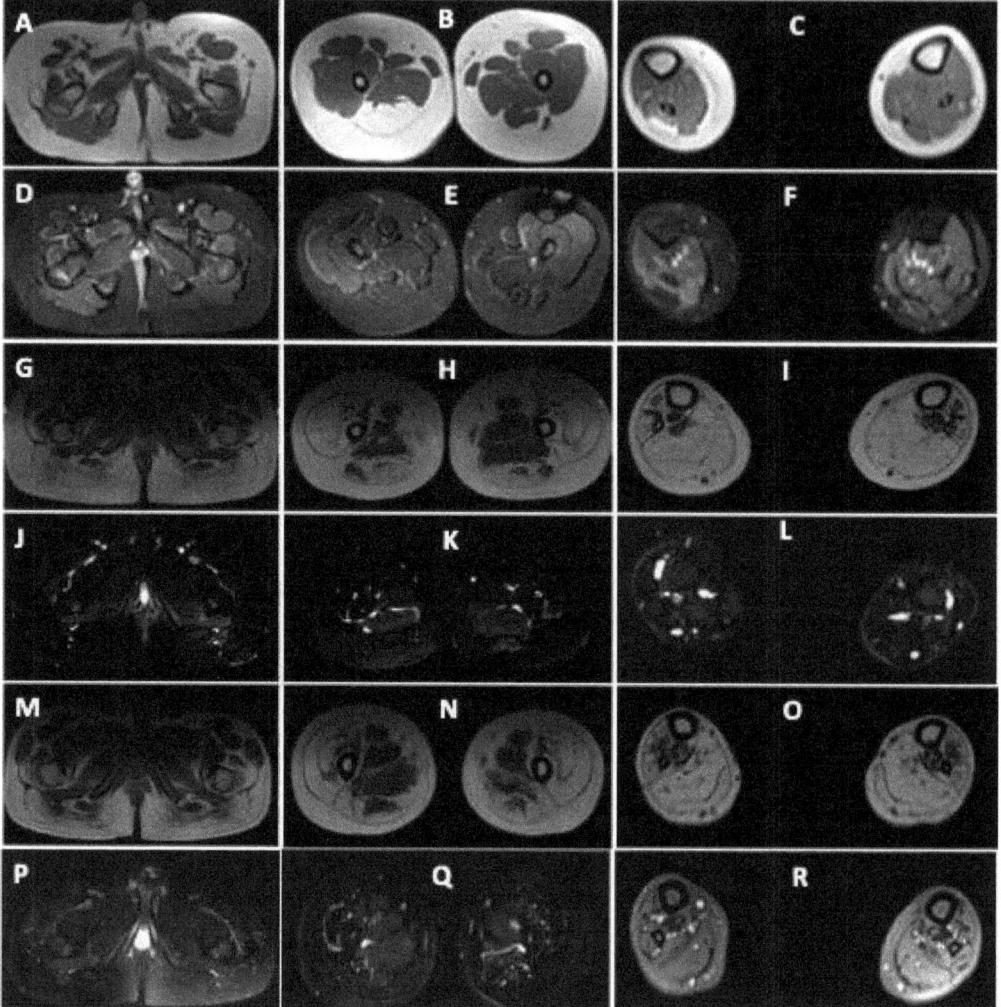

Figure 2. Muscle MRI images of patients with DA5D: (**A–F**) muscle MRI images of patient 1: axial T1-weighted sections at the level of the (**A**) pelvis, (**B**) midthigh, and (**C**) midleg reveal volume loss with fatty replacement, most pronounced in bilateral tensor fascia lata (Mercuri Grade 3), right semimembranosus (Grade 3), semitendinosus (Grade 3), bilateral biceps femoris (Grade 2b). Grade 2a fatty replacement is seen in the lateral compartment of the right leg and gastrocnemius. Axial fat-saturated T2-weighted sections at the level of the (**D**) pelvis, (**E**) midthigh, and (**F**) midleg reveal no edema; (**G–L**) MRI images of patient 2 and (**M–R**) of patient 3: axial T1-weighted sections at the level of the (**G,M**) pelvis, (**H,N**) midthigh, and (**I,O**) midleg reveal volume loss with fatty replacement, most pronounced in bilateral gluteus maximus (Mercuri Grade 3), vasti (Grade3), rectus femoris (Grade 2a), semimembranosus (Grade 2b), semitendinosus (Grade 2b), biceps femoris (Grade 2b). Grade 2b fatty replacement is seen in the anterior, lateral, and deep posterior compartments of the legs. The superficial posterior compartment of both legs reveals Grade 4 atrophy with fatty replacement. Axial fat-saturated T2-weighted sections at the level of the (**J,P**) pelvis, (**K,Q**) midthigh, and (**L,R**) midleg reveal no fluid signal.

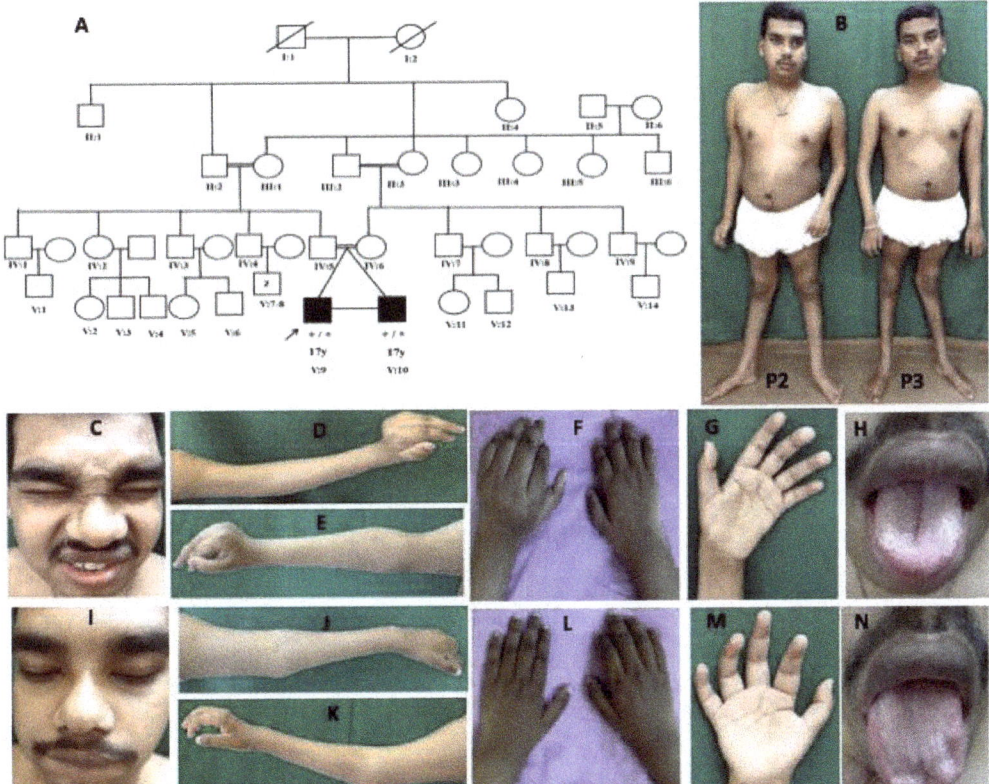

Figure 3. Pedigree and clinical images of patients 2 and 3 with DA5D: (**A**) pedigree of family 2; (**B**) clinical photograph of patients 2 and 3 showing contractures at elbows, fingers, hyperlordosis, and hyperextension at the knee; (**C–H**) patient 2: (**C**) facial weakness, hypertelorism, bulbous nose; (**D–G**) Left > Right contracture at elbows, wrist in extension and fingers at metacarpophalangeal (MCP) and interphalangeal joint (IPJ), and (**H**) furrowed tongue; (**I–N**) patient 3: (**I**) facial weakness, hypertelorism, bulbous nose; (**J–M**) Right > Left contracture at elbows, wrist in extension, and fingers at MCP and IPJ, and (**N**) atrophy of tongue.

There was diffuse atrophy of limb muscles with hypotonia, weakness of all limbs (distal > proximal, MRC grade: shoulder (4), elbow (3), wrist (3), fingers (3), hip (4), knee (4), ankle (0)), and absent tendon reflexes. A clinical diagnosis of hereditary motor neuropathy with unusual contractures was considered. At the last follow-up (20 years of age) during July 2021, seizure frequency had reduced, and the patient needed more support to ambulate.

Patient 3 is the monozygotic twin of patient 2. He was born at term by normal delivery with a birth weight of 1.75 kg (<5th percentile) and had normal perinatal history. He presented with delay in motor milestones, started walking independently at 6 years of age with altered high stepping gait, and had slowly progressive weakness and wasting of limbs. There was no history of seizures or intellectual disability. On examination, he had hypertelorism, tented upper lip, white hairlock, bulbous nose, mild tongue furrowing, normal fundus, and extraocular movements, mild bifacial weakness, asymmetric contractures at fingers (metacarpophalangeal and interphalangeal joints), wrist in extension, and elbow with knee hyperextensibility and pes cavus (Figure 3). There was diffuse atrophy of limb muscles with hypotonia, weakness of limbs (distal > proximal MRC grade: shoulder (4), elbow (4), wrist (4), fingers (3), hip (4), knee (3), ankle (3)), and absent tendon reflexes. At the last follow-up (20 years of age) during July 2021, the clinical condition was stationary.

Investigations in the twins revealed normal creatine kinase, hepatic, renal, and thyroid function tests. Serum lactate was 41.2 (patient 2) and 26.3 (patient 3) (reference range: 4.5 to 20 mg/dl), while ammonia, HbA1c, homocysteine, plasma amino acids, and acylcarnitine profile were normal in both. Nerve conduction studies (NCS) in both revealed normal sensory nerve conductions (right median, ulnar and sural), impaired motor conduction studies of the right median, and ulnar with reduced amplitude, normal latency, and conduction velocities (Table 1). The right common peroneal nerve was inexcitable. EMG of the tibialis anterior showed fibrillations, positive sharp waves with high amplitude polyphasic motor unit action potentials (MUAPs) with mildly reduced recruitment. Similarly, abductor digiti minimi (ADM) showed evidence of high amplitude polyphasic MUAPs, suggestive of a neurogenic pattern. Repetitive nerve stimulation at 3Hz did not reveal a significant decrement response from orbicularis oculi, trapezius, and ADM muscles.

Table 1. Nerve conduction studies of patients 2 and 3.

	Parameters	Patient 2	Patient 3
Motor conduction study	Distal Latency(ms)/CMAP(mV)/MNCV (m/s)		
	Median	3.84/1.73/49.3	3.5/1.32/60.6
	Ulnar	3.86/0.8/49.7	2.25/2.61/61.8
	CPN	absent	absent
Sensory conduction study	Onset Latency(ms)/SNAP(uV)/SNCV (m/s)		
	Median	3.04/12.8/52.6	2.86/20.1/55.9
	Ulnar	2.84/10.76/50	2.12/15.4/56.9
	Sural	3.02/8.79/53	3.06/11/45.8

ADM: abductor digiti minimi, CMAP: compound motor action potential, CPN: common peroneal nerve, MNCV: motor nerve conduction velocity, NA: not available, SNCV: sensory nerve conduction velocity.

Muscle MRI in both revealed volume loss with fatty replacement, most pronounced in bilateral gluteus maximus, vasti, rectus femoris, hamstrings, and all muscles of the anterior, lateral, and posterior compartments of legs. Hip adductors and sartorius were spared (Figure 2).

Brain MRI in patient 2 revealed focal encephalomalacia with adjacent gliosis in bilateral parieto-occipital regions with a paucity of white matter, thinning of body, and splenium of corpus callosum suggestive of hypoxic-ischemic injury. Brain MRI in patient 3 revealed symmetric T2/FLAIR hyperintensities in bilateral parieto-occipital and corticospinal tracts.

Genetic Results

Trios NGS performed in both families identified *ECEL1* homozygous disease-causing variants in patients 1, 2, and 3 from families 1 and 2, respectively. Patient 1 had a novel homozygous missense variant in exon 2 of *ECEL1* (NM_004826.4): c.602T > C (p.Met201Thr), in the extracellular Peptidase M13 domain (Uniprot). The variant is present in heterozygous form in both parents and is not reported in the general population (Gnomad frequency: 0). In silico predictions determined the variant as damaging/pathogenic, and it is classified as "likely pathogenic" as per ACMG criteria (PM1, PM2, PP2, PP3).

Patients 2 and 3 were identified to have a novel homozygous missense variant in exon 2 of *ECEL1*: c.83C > T (p.Ala28Val), which is located in the proximal cytoplasmic domain. While the variant is segregated as heterozygous in both parents, it is present with low frequency in the general population (Gnomad MAF: 0.005%; Heterozygotes −3; Homozygotes-nil). The in silico predictions were pathogenic by SIFT and additional analysis by human splicing finder (HSF—https://hsf.genomnis.com/home, accessed on 15 April 2021) [9] showed "Potential alteration of splicing due to activation of a cryptic donor site". Based on ACMG criteria, c.83C > T (p.Ala28Val) has been classified as "likely pathogenic" (PM1, PM2, PP2, PP3).

4. Discussion

Arthrogryposis multiplex congenita is a heterogeneous condition caused by a myriad of disorders including aneuploidy syndromes, skeletal dysplasias, multiple congenital anomaly syndromes, and neuromuscular diseases [1,2]. Among these, a group of disorders characterized mainly, but not exclusively, by abnormalities of the distal limbs were described as distal arthrogryposes (DAs) in 1982, by Hall et al. [2]. Subsequently, DA has been defined as an inherited primary limb malformation disorder characterized by congenital contractures of two or more different body areas and without primary neurologic and/or muscle disease that affects limb function [2]. Major diagnostic criteria include ulnar deviation, camptodactyly (or pseudocamptodactyly), hypoplastic and/or absent flexion creases, and or overriding fingers, talipes equinovarus, calcaneo-valgus deformities, vertical talus, and/or metatarsus varus [2].

Most DAs are autosomal dominant disorders caused by genes encoding proteins related to the muscle contraction apparatus [2,3]. However, distal arthrogryposis type 5D is autosomal recessive and is usually caused by biallelic mutations in *ECEL1* [3].

Distal arthrogryposis type 5 D is characterized by a wide array of clinical features including (i) musculoskeletal with foot deformities, finger contractures, and limited movement of proximal joints, recurrent hip dislocation, webbing of fingers and neck, scoliosis, kyphosis, muscle atrophy, and weakness; (ii) ophthalmological with asymmetric ptosis, strabismus, refractive errors, and ophthalmoplegia; (iii) facial with arched eyebrows, bulbous upturned nose, micrognathia, small mouth, reduced facial expression, cleft palate and tongue atrophy; (iv) others including speech difficulties, nasal voice, short stature, short neck, cryptorchidism, pterygia, faint palmar creases, and respiratory dysfunction [3–5,10–19]. Progressive scoliosis and weakness of limbs have been reported on long-term follow-up of these patients [11]. Consanguineous parentage with a history of reduced fetal movements may give an additional clue to the diagnosis. The fetal movements were normal in our patients. Characteristics of patients reported in the literature and our patients with DA5D are summarized in Table 2.

In addition to features described earlier, our patients had additional features of white hairlock, proptosis, prominent knee hyperextensibility, and areflexia, thus further expanding the clinical spectrum of this disorder. However, distal interphalangeal joint hyperlaxity and areflexia have been reported in a few patients [4]. Global development delay, recurrent seizures, and mental subnormality in patient 2 can possibly be attributed to birth asphyxia and brain injury.

ECEL1 encodes endothelin-converting enzyme-like 1, a type II integral transmembrane zinc metalloprotease, similar to the endothelin-converting enzyme (ECE) structurally but functionally different, as *ECEL1* does not cleave ECE substrates [5,10]. Mouse studies have shown that damage-induced neuronal endopeptidase (DINE; rodent homolog of *ECEL1*) is significantly upregulated in both the peripheral and central nervous systems. *ECEL1* is essential for the final axonal arborization of motor nerves in the diaphragm, limb skeletal muscles, and for the formation of proper neuromuscular junctions (NMJs) during prenatal development [10]. Failure of formation and maturation of the embryonic neuromuscular end plate and NMJs leads to early and sustained lack of movement in utero causing pterygia, webs, and contractures [10]. Further, the twins had prominent foot drop mimicking a progressive motor neuropathy, which was also corroborated the severe motor axonopathy. These features have not been reported earlier in English literature.

Table 2. Comparison of clinical features of this study with previous studies.

Clinical Features	McMillin et al.	Dieterich et al.	Shaheen et al.	Shaaban et al.	Patil et al.	Barnett et al.	Bayram et al.	Hamzeh et al.	Ullmann et al.	Stattin et al.	Umair et al.	Jin et al.	Alei et al.	Total	Present Study
Year of study	2013	2013	2014	2014	2014	2014	2016	2017	2018	2018	2019	2020	2021		2021
Number of patients	9	10	9	2	1	2	4	1	7	1	2	1	2	51	3
Consanguinity	2/9	9/10	9/9	2/2	1/1	0/2	4/4	1/1	4/7	1/1	2/2	0/1	1/2	36/51	3/3
Male:Female	5:4	5:5	3:6	1:1	0:1	1:1	3:1	1:0	2:5	1:0	2:0	1:0	0:2	25:26	3:0
Contractures															
Foot or toe contractures and/or deformity	9/9	9/10	4/9	2/2	1/1	2/2	3/3	1/1	6/7	1/1	2/2	0/1	2/2	42/50	3/3
Ankle	9/9	NA	NA	0/2	NA	2/2	NA	NA	6/7	1/1	2/2	NA	NA	20/23	1/3
Knee	8/9	10/10	5/5	2/2	1/1	2/2	1/1	1/1	7/7	1/1	2/2	1/1	2/2	43/44	1/3
Hip dislocation and/or limitation of movement	9/9	9/9	6/9	0/2	1/1	2/2	3/3	1/1	5/7	1/1	NA	NA	1/2	38/46	1/3
Hand and/or finger	9/9	10/10	9/9	2/2	1/1	2/2	4/4	1/1	7/7	1/1	2/2	1/1	2/2	51/51	3/3
Wrist	9/9	NA	1/1	2/2	NA	2/2	NA	NA	2/7	1/1	NA	1/1	2/2	20/25	2/3
Elbow	5/5	3/7	1/1	0/2	1/1	2/2	1/1	1/1	3/7	1/1	2/2	1/1	1/2	22/33	3/3
Shoulder	6/6	2/8	1/1	1/2	0/1	0/2	NA	NA	4/7	1/1	NA	NA	2/2	18/31	0/3
Neck	4/4	NA	NA	2/2	NA	1/2	NA	NA	NA	1/1	0/2	NA	2/2	9/10	0/3
Webbed neck	3/8	NA	NA	2/2	NA	NA	NA	1/1	2/7	1/1	NA	NA	NA	9/21	0/3
Ptosis	8/9	7/10	6/9	1/2	1/1	2/2	1/1	1/1	5/7	1/1	2/2	1/1	1/2	37/48	1/3
Strabismus	1/1	1/10	3/9	2/2	0/1	NA	NA	NA	1/7	NA	2/2	1/1	1/2	12/35	1/3
Ophthalmoplegia	0/9	1/10	NA	2/2	0/1	NA	NA	NA	0/7	NA	0/2	NA	1/2	4/33	0/3
Bulbous nose	9/9	NA	2/2	2/2	1/1	NA	2/2	NA	NA	1/1	NA	NA	NA	17/17	2/3
Reduced facial movements	1/9	3/7	NA	2/2	NA	NA	NA	NA	5/7	1/1	NA	1/1	1/2	14/29	3/3
Micrognathia/small mouth	8/9	3/10	1/1	2/2	1/1	1/1	2/2	1/1	4/7	1/1	0/2	NA	2/2	26/39	1/3
Cleft palate	1/1	1/1	NA	NA	1/1	NA	NA	NA	2/7	1/1	0/2	1/1	0/2	7/16	0/3
Tongue atrophy/furrowing	NA	7/7	NA	NA	1/1	0/2	NA	1/1	4/5	1/1	0/2	NA	1/2	15/21	2/3
Short neck	4/7	10/10	NA	2/2	1/1	NA	NA	1/1	NA	NA	NA	NA	2/2	19/22	0/3
Speech Abnormalities	NA	5/5	NA	NA	NA	NA	NA	1/1	NA	NA	2/2	NA	1/2	8/9	1/3
Scoliosis	2/9	7/10	2/9	2/2	1/1	NA	1/1	1/1	3/7	1/1	0/2	NA	2/2	21/44	1/3
Hyperlordosis	NA	9/9	NA	1/2	0/1	NA	NA	NA	4/7	1/1	NA	NA	2/2	12/14	0/3
Muscle atrophy	NA	10/10	NA	2/2	1/1	NA	NA	1/1	4/7	1/1	1/2	NA	1/2	21/26	3/3

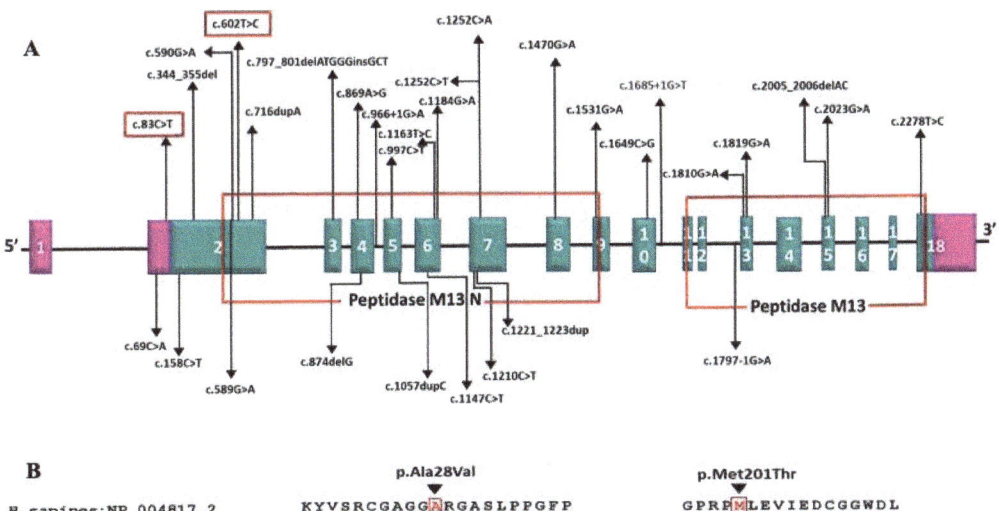

Figure 4. (**A**) Schematic representation of the variations identified in the *ECEL1* gene with corresponding exons and protein domains. The 18 exons of *ECEL1* (NM_004826.4) are represented as boxes with respective exon numbers. Regions of exons coding for UTRs are marked in violet color at the ends. The protein domains are according to the Uniprot database. The novel variant found in our is study is marked in the box. The size of exons /introns is not represented at scale; (**B**) amino acid conservation at positions 28 and 201 across species.

DA5D is caused by recessive mutations in the *ECEL1* gene [3,4]. We identified homozygous novel missense variants c.602T > C (p.Met201Thr) and c.83C > T (p.Ala28Val) in exon 2 of *ECEL1* gene in families 1 and 2, respectively. The c.602T > C (p.Met201Thr) variant affects the crucial Peptidase M13 extracellular domain where all the previous disease-causing missense mutations have been reported. Two missense mutations affecting a nearby codon 197 (p.Gly197Asp and p.Gly197Ser) have been reported in DA5D patients of European ancestry by McMillin et al. and Ullmann et al., respectively [3,11] (Figure 4).

These patients had a similar phenotype of fixed contractures at birth and progressive weakness. However, Ullmann et al. reported a consanguineous family with two affected siblings and another affected cousin who had identical p.Gly197Ser homozygous mutation with long-term follow up and disease progression [11]. The elder female sibling in the family did not have ptosis and had additional temporomandibular contractures not reported in other patients [11]. Interestingly, our patient 1 also had trismus due to temporomandibular joint contractures. Ullmann et al. also reported that ambulation is preserved in patients even into the third decade with slowly progressive muscle weakness [11]. Mild learning difficulties and exercise intolerance were some of the unusual findings identified in the elder sibling on long-term follow-up [11]. However, brain MRI was not performed, and there was no evidence of NMJ dysfunction in EMG study [11]. Likewise, our patients 1 and 3 had a stable nonprogressive course and were independently ambulant at 15 and 20 years, respectively. However, patient 3 had a significant motor disability and remains status quo.

In patients 2 and 3 (twin siblings affected in family 2), the c.83C > T (p.Ala28Val) variant was identified in the proximal cytoplasmic domain. Based on literature evidence and ClinVar-reported mutations, only two nonsense mutations c.69C > A (p.Cys23Ter) and c.33C > G (p.Tyr11Ter) associated with DA5D phenotype have been reported previously in the cytoplasmic domain of *ECEL1* [10,20]. The phenotypic pattern of fixed contractures at birth with slowly progressive weakness reported with proximal nonsense mutations was not dissimilar to those with mutations in the downstream extracellular domain, suggesting a common pathomechanism irrespective of location and type of mutation. The mutation c.83C > T (p.Ala28Val) identified in our study is the first disease-causing missense variant affecting the proximal cytoplasmic domain of *ECEL1*. Additional in silico analysis by human splicing finder (HSF) predicted that c.83C > T can cause significant alteration of wild type splicing mechanism by activating a cryptic donor splice site in exon 2 and also altering the ratio of exonic-splicing enhancers and silencers (ESE/ESS). While this can result in partial deletion of exon 2 and/or exon skipping, additional RNA analysis might be required to confirm the impact on protein expression [9]. We admit that the lack of functional validation for c.83C > T (p.Ala28Val) is a limitation for this study due to the nonavailability of tissue samples from patients. Nevertheless, these in silico predictions suggest a loss of function mechanism similar to previous nonsense mutations identified in the proximal cytoplasmic domain [10,20].

There are only a few reports on muscle MRI in patients with DA5D [4,11]. Severe fatty infiltration of thighs affecting the biceps femoris, sartorius and vastus lateralis, extensor digitorum longus, and asymmetric involvement of distal leg muscles with sparing of rectus femoris and gracilis has been reported [4,11]. All three patients in the current study underwent muscle MRI. Diffuse fatty infiltration was observed involving hamstrings and gastrocnemius in all, and extensive fatty infiltration of gluteus maximus, quadriceps, anterior, lateral, and posterior compartments of legs was also observed in the two monozygotic twins. This further implies a wider spectrum of disease involvement. It is interesting to note that the severity of muscle weakness was different in patients 2 and 3, but the severity of MRI findings was almost identical.

5. Conclusions

Distal arthrogryposis type 5D is a very rare autosomal recessive disorder caused by mutations in *ECEL1* characterized predominantly by distal contractures. Being an autosomal recessive disorder, it has implications in genetic counseling. Here, we described three patients with novel mutations, and additional clinical and imaging features compared with earlier descriptions, thus expanding the clinical, imaging, and molecular spectrum of the *ECEL1* mutations and associated DA5D.

Supplementary Materials: The following are available online at https://www.mdpi.com/article/10.3390/children8100909/s1, Table S1: Coverage of arthrogryposis and congenital myasthenic syndrome panel genes in patient 1, Table S2: Coverage of Charcot-Marie-Tooth and other sensory neuropathies and arthrogryposis & congenital myasthenic syndrome genes in patient 2 and 3.

Author Contributions: Conceptualization, A.N.; methodology, K.P.; software, genetic analysis, G.A.; validation, G.A.; formal analysis, K.P. and G.A.; investigation, V.P.-K., P.P. and K.K.; data curation, M.B. and G.U.; writing—original draft preparation: A.H., S.V. and S.N.; writing—review and editing: A.N, M.B. and H.L.; visualization: A.N.; supervision: A.N. and K.P. All authors have read and agreed to the published version of the manuscript.

Funding: This research received no external funding.

Institutional Review Board Statement: The study was conducted according to the guidelines of the Declaration of Helsinki, and this retrospective study was approved by the Institutional Ethics Committee of NIMHANS (NIMHANS/IEC/2020-21 approved on 1 September 2020).

Informed Consent Statement: Written informed consent has been obtained from the patient(s) to publish this paper.

Data Availability Statement: The clinical and raw genetic data are available for review with the corresponding author and available on request.

Conflicts of Interest: H Lochmüller receives support from the Canadian Institutes of Health Research (Foundation Grant FDN-167281), the Canadian Institutes of Health Research and Muscular Dystrophy Canada (Network Catalyst Grant for NMD4C), the Canada Foundation for Innovation (CFI-JELF 38412), and the Canada Research Chairs program (Canada Research Chair in Neuromuscular Genomics and Health, 950-232279). The other authors declare no conflict of interest.

References

1. Hall, J.G. Arthrogryposis (multiple congenital contractures): Diagnostic approach to etiology, classification, genetics, and general principles. *Eur. J. Med. Genet.* **2014**, *57*, 464–472. [CrossRef] [PubMed]
2. Bamshad, M.; Jorde, L.B.; Carey, J.C. A revised and extended classification of the distal arthrogryposes. *Am. J. Med. Genet.* **1996**, *65*, 277–281. [CrossRef]
3. McMillin, M.J.; Below, J.E.; Shively, K.M.; Beck, A.E.; Gildersleeve, H.I.; Pinner, J.; Gogola, G.R.; Hecht, J.T.; Grange, D.K.; Harris, D.J.; et al. Mutations in ECEL1 cause distal arthrogryposis type 5D. *Am. J. Hum. Genet.* **2013**, *92*, 150–156. [CrossRef] [PubMed]
4. Dieterich, K.; Quijano-Roy, S.; Monnier, N.; Beck, A.E.; Gildersleeve, H.I.; Pinner, J.; Gogola, G.R.; Hecht, J.T.; Grange, D.K.; Harris, D.J.; et al. The neuronal endopeptidase ECEL1 is associated with a distinct form of recessive distal arthrogryposis. *Hum. Mol. Genet.* **2013**, *22*, 1483–1492. [CrossRef] [PubMed]
5. Umair, M.; Khan, A.; Hayat, A.; Abbas, S.; Asiri, A.; Younus, M.; Amin, W.; Nawaz, S.; Khan, S.; Malik, E.; et al. Biallelic Missense Mutation in the *ECEL1* Underlies Distal Arthrogryposis Type 5 (DA5D). *Front. Pediatr.* **2019**, *7*, 343. [CrossRef] [PubMed]
6. Li, H.; Durbin, R. Fast and accurate long-read alignment with Burrows-Wheeler transform. *Bioinformatics* **2010**, *26*, 589–595. [CrossRef] [PubMed]
7. McKenna, A.; Hanna, M.; Banks, E.; Sivachenko, A.; Cibulskis, K.; Kernytsky, A.; Garimella, K.; Altshuler, D.; Gabriel, S.; Daly, M.; et al. The Genome Analysis Toolkit: A MapReduce framework for analyzing next-generation DNA sequencing data. *Genome. Res.* **2010**, *20*, 1297–1303. [CrossRef] [PubMed]
8. Richards, S.; Aziz, N.; Bale, S.; Bick, D.; Das, S.; Gastier-Foster, J.; Grody, W.W.; Hegde, M.; Lyon, E.; Spector, E.; et al. Standards and guidelines for the interpretation of sequence variants: A joint consensus recommendation of the American College of Medical Genetics and Genomics and the Association for Molecular Pathology. *Genet. Med.* **2015**, *17*, 405–424. [CrossRef] [PubMed]
9. Desmet, F.O.; Hamroun, D.; Lalande, M.; Collod-Béroud, G.; Claustres, M.; Béroud, C. Human Splicing Finder: An online bioinformatics tool to predict splicing signals. *Nucleic Acids Res.* **2009**, *37*, e67. [CrossRef] [PubMed]
10. Jin, J.Y.; Liu, D.Y.; Jiao, Z.J.; Dong, Y.; Li, J.; Xiang, R. The Novel Compound Heterozygous Mutations of *ECEL1* Identified in a Family with Distal Arthrogryposis Type 5D. *Biomed. Res. Int.* **2020**, *2020*, 2149342. [CrossRef] [PubMed]
11. Ullmann, U.; D'Argenzio, L.; Mathur, S.; Whyte, T.; Quinlivan, R.; Longman, C.; Farrugia, M.E.; Manzur, A.; Willis, T.; Jungbluth, H.; et al. ECEL1 gene related contractural syndrome: Long-term follow-up and update on clinical and pathological aspects. *Neuromuscul. Disord.* **2018**, *28*, 741–749. [CrossRef] [PubMed]
12. Shaheen, R.; Al-Owain, M.; Khan, A.O.; Zaki, M.S.; Hossni, H.A.; Al-Tassan, R.; Eyaid, W.; Alkuraya, F.S. Identification of three novel ECEL1 mutations in three families with distal arthrogryposis type 5D. *Clin. Genet.* **2014**, *85*, 568–572. [CrossRef] [PubMed]
13. Shaaban, S.; Duzcan, F.; Yildirim, C.; Chan, W.M.; Andrews, C.; Akarsu, N.A.; Engle, E.C. Expanding the phenotypic spectrum of ECEL1-related congenital contracture syndromes. *Clin. Genet.* **2014**, *85*, 562–567. [CrossRef] [PubMed]
14. Patil, S.J.; Rai, G.K.; Bhat, V.; Ramesh, V.A.; Nagarajaram, H.A.; Matalia, J.; Phadke, S.R. Distal arthrogryposis type 5D with a novel ECEL1 gene mutation. *Am. J. Med. Genet. A* **2014**, *164A*, 2857–2862. [CrossRef] [PubMed]
15. Barnett, C.P.; Todd, E.J.; Ong, R.; Davis, M.R.; Atkinson, V.; Allcock, R.; Laing, N.; Ravenscroft, G. Distal arthrogryposis type 5D with novel clinical features and compound heterozygous mutations in ECEL1. *Am. J. Med. Genet. A* **2014**, *164A*, 1846–1849. [CrossRef] [PubMed]
16. Bayram, Y.; Karaca, E.; CobanAkdemir, Z.; Yilmaz, E.O.; Tayfun, G.A.; Aydin, H.; Torun, D.; Bozdogan, S.T.; Gezdirici, A.; Isikay, S. Molecular etiology of arthrogryposis in multiple families of mostly Turkish origin. *J. Clin. Investig.* **2016**, *126*, 762–778. [CrossRef] [PubMed]
17. Hamzeh, A.R.; Nair, P.; Mohamed, M.; Saif, F.; Tawfiq, N.; Khalifa, M.; Al-Ali, M.T.; Bastaki, F. A Novel Variant in the Endothelin-Converting Enzyme-Like 1 (ECEL1) Gene in an Emirati Child. *Med. Princ. Pract.* **2017**, *26*, 195–198. [CrossRef] [PubMed]
18. Stattin, E.L.; Johansson, J.; Gudmundsson, S.; Ameur, A.; Lundberg, S.; Bondeson, M.L.; Wilbe, M. A novel ECEL1 mutation expands the phenotype of distal arthrogryposis multiplex congenita type 5D to include pretibial vertical skin creases. *Am. J. Med. Genet. A* **2018**, *176*, 1405–1410. [CrossRef] [PubMed]
19. Alesi, V.; Sessini, F.; Genovese, S.; Calvieri, G.; Sallicandro, E.; Ciocca, L.; Mingoia, M.; Novelli, A.; Moi, P. A New Intronic Variant in ECEL1 in Two Patients with Distal Arthrogryposis Type 5D. *Int. J. Mol. Sci.* **2021**, *22*, 2106. [CrossRef] [PubMed]
20. Laquérriere, A.; Maluenda, J.; Camus, A.; Fontenas, L.; Dieterich, K.; Nolent, F.; Zhou, J.; Monnier, N.; Latour, P.; Gentil, D. Mutations in CNTNAP1 and ADCY6 are responsible for severe arthrogryposis multiplex congenita with axoglial defects. *Hum. Mol. Genet.* **2014**, *23*, 2279–2289. [CrossRef] [PubMed]

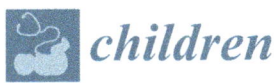

Case Report

Neuralgic Amyotrophy with Concomitant Hereditary Neuropathy with Liability to Pressure Palsy as a Cause of Dropped Shoulder in a Child after Human Papillomavirus Vaccination: A Case Report

Hye-Chan Ahn [1], Do-Hoon Kim [2], Chul-Hyun Cho [3], Jun-Chul Byun [4] and Jang-Hyuk Cho [1,*]

1. Department of Rehabilitation Medicine, Keimyung University Dongsan Hospital, Keimyung University School of Medicine, Daegu 42601, Korea; plokij36@naver.com
2. Department of Laboratory Medicine, Keimyung University Dongsan Hospital, Keimyung University School of Medicine, Daegu 42601, Korea; kdh@dsmc.or.kr
3. Department of Orthopedic Surgery, Keimyung University Dongsan Hospital, Keimyung University School of Medicine, Daegu 42601, Korea; oscho5362@dsmc.or.kr
4. Department of Pediatrics, Keimyung University Dongsan Hospital, Keimyung University School of Medicine, Daegu 42601, Korea; goodpeddr@naver.com
* Correspondence: rehacho@hanmail.net; Tel.: +82-53-258-7912

Abstract: Hereditary neuropathy with liability to pressure palsy (HNPP) makes nerves increasingly susceptible to mechanical pressure at entrapment sites. Neuralgic amyotrophy (NA) can cause sudden regional weakness following events to which the patient is immunologically predisposed, such as vaccination. However, NA related to human papilloma virus (HPV) vaccination is seldom reported. We describe the case of a child with NA as the cause of a dropped shoulder following the administration of the HPV vaccine. Underlying asymptomatic HNPP was confirmed in this patient based on the electrodiagnostic findings and genetic analysis. We speculate that HPV vaccination elicited an immune-mediated inflammatory response, resulting in NA. Our patient with pre-existing HNPP might be vulnerable to the occurrence of an immune-mediated NA, which caused the dropped shoulder.

Keywords: brachial plexus neuritis; hereditary sensory and motor neuropathy; paralysis; vaccination; pediatrics

1. Introduction

Hereditary neuropathy with liability to pressure palsy (HNPP) is a rare autosomal dominant peripheral nerve disorder [1]. Clinical features include painless, recurrent, and transient weakness at entrapment sites or susceptible pressure points [2]. The frequently involved patterns are similar to those seen in entrapment neuropathy; however, brachial plexus involvement is uncommon [1,2].

Neuralgic amyotrophy (NA) is a markedly underdiagnosed or misdiagnosed peripheral nerve disease due to the heterogeneity of clinical appearance [3]. It represents a sudden onset of paralysis, atrophy, and sensory deficits in the shoulder region with a preceding episode of severe pain [4]. Although the exact pathophysiology of NA has not yet been established, it is presumably associated with inflammatory autoimmune pathophysiology [3,4]. Vaccination is less commonly known to be related to the occurrence of NA [4,5].

This study was approved by our institutional review board (IRB number: 2021-01-079). Written informed consent was obtained from the patient's legal guardian. This report describes the case of a female child who presented with a dropped shoulder due to NA following administration of the human papillomavirus (HPV) vaccine. We found that

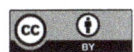

she also had underlying HNPP during the diagnostic process. There are currently no published cases of NA with concomitant HNPP occurring after HPV vaccination. HPV vaccination is suspected to elicit an immune-mediated inflammatory response, resulting in NA. Patients with pre-existing HNPP, although asymptomatic, might have potential vulnerability to the occurrence of an immune-mediated NA, thus causing symptoms, such as dropped shoulder.

2. Case Report

A 12-year-old female child received her first dose of Cervarix (GSK, Brentford, UK) vaccination for HPV prophylaxis in the left deltoid muscle. Five days after vaccination, the child complained of a sudden onset of painless dropped shoulder on the left side. She denied any history of trauma, notable physical exercise, or previous medical illness. No adverse events had occurred following the suggested pediatric immunization program and she had not been vaccinated for coronavirus disease 2019 (COVID-19). The patient's parents denied any family history of notable genetic diseases. On initial physical examination, there was Medical Research Council (MRC) grade 2 weakness of the shoulder abductor and flexor muscles and grade 3 weakness of the internal and external rotator muscles without atrophy. The sensation of the left upper lateral limb was altered on light touch. Deep tendon reflexes were normal, and no upper motor neuron lesion signs were observed.

Laboratory findings—including C-reactive protein, erythrocyte sedimentation rate, creatine kinase, antinuclear antibody, rheumatoid factor, and anti-GM1 ganglioside antibodies—were negative. We have also excluded infectious neuritis, including human immunodeficiency virus infection and Lyme disease. Magnetic resonance imaging (MRI) of the brain, cervical spine, and brachial plexus performed one week after symptom onset revealed no abnormal findings. Nerve conduction studies revealed the absence of the left lateral antebrachial cutaneous sensory nerve action potential (SNAP) and decreased amplitude in left axillary compound motor action potential (CMAP). It also showed generalized demyelinating polyneuropathy, including the following signs: slowing of the bilateral median, bilateral ulnar, bilateral common peroneal, and bilateral tibial nerve conduction velocity; prolonged distal latency of bilateral median SNAP; and borderline distal latency of bilateral median, bilateral ulnar, and bilateral common peroneal CMAP close to the upper limit of normal (Table 1). Needle electromyography showed active denervation potentials of the left supraspinatus, deltoid, and brachioradialis muscles. It also showed decreased motor unit recruitment in the left shoulder girdle muscles. This electrodiagnostic evaluation revealed left brachial plexopathy predominantly involving the upper trunk with generalized demyelinating polyneuropathy.

Table 1. Nerve conduction study results at presentation.

Nerve	Recording Site	Latency (ms) [Normal Value]	Amplitude (μV and mV) [Normal Value]	Velocity (m/s) [Normal Value]
Sensory				
Rt. median	Digit-2	3.15 [$\leq$3.5]	26.5 [$\geq$20]	
Lt. median	Digit-2	3.50 [$\leq$3.5]	19.7 [$\geq$20]	
Rt. ulnar	Digit-5	2.75 [$\leq$3.2]	29.6 [$\geq$17]	
Lt. ulnar	Digit-5	2.85 [$\leq$3.2]	26.5 [$\geq$17]	
Rt. sural	Lat. malleolus	2.55 [$\leq$4.2]	11.7 [$\geq$6]	
Lt. sural	Lat. malleolus	2.70 [$\leq$4.2]	9.3 [$\geq$6]	

Table 1. Cont.

Nerve	Recording Site	Latency (ms) [Normal Value]	Amplitude (μV and mV) [Normal Value]	Velocity (m/s) [Normal Value]
Rt. sup. peroneal	Foot	3.05 [≤4.4]	9.3 [≥6]	
Lt. sup. peroneal	Foot	3.30 [≤4.4]	5.9 [≥6]	
Rt. MAC	Forearm	1.90 [≤3.2]	10.7 [≥5]	
Lt. MAC	Forearm	1.90 [≤3.2]	8.5 [≥5]	
Rt. LAC	Forearm	1.70 [≤3.0]	25.7 [≥10]	
Lt. LAC	Forearm	No response		
Motor				
Rt. median	APB	4.00 [≤4.1]	12.1 [≥5.5]	47.5 [≥50]
Lt. median	APB	4.15 [≤4.1]	9.8 [≥5.5]	44.7 [≥50]
Rt. ulnar	ADM	3.15 [≤3.1]	11.1 [≥5.9]	47.5 [≥52]
Lt. ulnar	ADM	3.05 [≤3.1]	10.7 [≥5.9]	45.8 [≥52]
Rt. common peroneal	EDB	5.25 [≤5.6]	4.2 [≥2.0]	40.6 [≥41]
Lt. common peroneal	EDB	5.35 [≤5.6]	3.8 [≥2.0]	37.2 [≥41]
Rt. tibial	AH	3.40 [≤5.4]	10.0 [≥4.6]	38.2 [≥42]
Lt. tibial	AH	3.55 [≤5.4]	9.9 [≥4.6]	39.0 [≥42]
Rt. axillary	Deltoid	2.25 [≤4.9]	12.3	
Lt. axillary	Deltoid	2.45 [≤4.9]	0.7	
Rt. musculocutaneous	Biceps	4.10 [≤5.7]	5.6	
Lt. musculocutaneous	Biceps	4.30 [≤5.7]	5.9	
Rt. suprascapular	SST	2.50 [≤3.7]	6.0	
Lt. suprascapular	SST	2.00 [≤3.7]	7.0	

MAC, medial antebrachial cutaneous nerve; LAC, lateral antebrachial cutaneous nerve; APB, abductor pollicis brevis; ADM, abductor digiti minimi; EDB, extensor digitorum brevis; AH, abductor hallucis; SST, supraspinatus.

Based on her medical history and the results of our evaluations, the patient was diagnosed with NA with peripheral polyneuropathy. Cerebrospinal fluid analysis to rule out acute or chronic inflammatory demyelinating polyneuropathy showed no abnormal findings. Genetic analysis was performed to identify the cause of hereditary polyneuropathy. Multiple ligation probe amplification (MLPA) was performed by probe mixes P033-B4 to detect copy number variations (CNVs) in the *PMP22* gene (MRC-Holland, Amsterdam, The Netherlands). Coffalyser.Net (MRC-Holland) was used for fragment analysis. The height ratio of the polymerase chain reaction (PCR)-derived fluorescence peaks was measured to quantify the amount of PCR products after normalization, and CNVs were identified when the ratio was <0.65 or >1.3. The MLPA revealed a contiguous heterozygous gene deletion of chromosome 17p11.2 that includes *COX10*, *PMP22*, and *TEKT3*, which confirmed the diagnosis of HNPP (Figure 1).

The patient received oral prednisolone for 10 days (40 mg/day for 5 days, the dose of which was then tapered for another 5 days) and underwent two courses of this treatment. Five months after the onset of symptoms, the patient recovered completely.

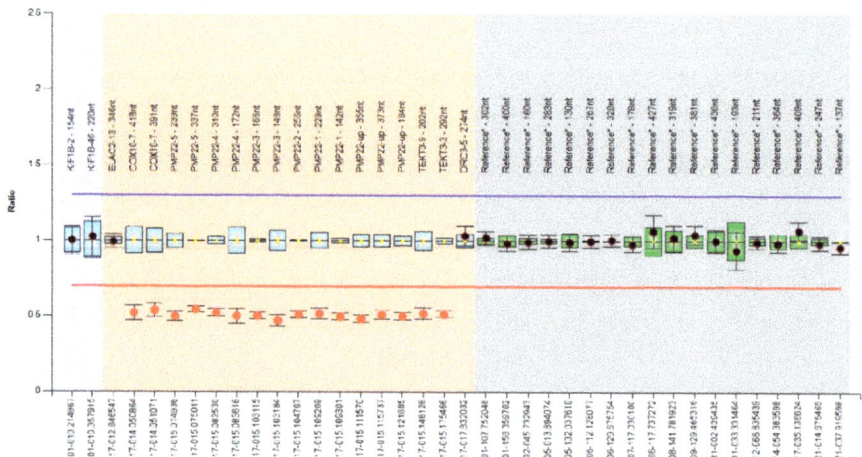

Figure 1. MLPA results of samples with contiguous gene deletion of chromosome 17p11.2 that included *COX10*, *PMP22*, and *TEKT3* in the bar chart generated using Coffalyser.Net. The x- and y-axes indicate the names of each MLPA probe and the peak ratio, respectively. The reference probe area is colored in gray. Deletions or duplications can be identified when the peak ratio was <0.65 (red line) or >1.3 (blue line), respectively. Exons with a reduced peak ratio (heterozygous deletion, between 0.40 and 0.65) are indicated with a red dot.

3. Discussion

HNPP is a hereditary neuropathy caused by deletion of the *PMP 22* gene that results in sausage-like focal thickening of the myelin sheath [1]. It is mostly diagnosed in early adulthood between 20 and 30 years of age, or if there is a family history [2]. HNPP is often triggered by physical activity, trivial compression, and negligible trauma that affects transient and recurrent focal neuropathy [2].

NA typically represents a preceding episode of severe pain before the sudden onset of paralysis [5]. However, some patients affected with NA complain of painless weakness in the region, such as in our case [4–6]. NA usually occurs between the age of 20 and 60 years. In addition, there is a biphasic peak of incidence in pediatric cases during the neonatal period and adolescence [4]. More than 50% of NA cases have a trigger event such as infection, vaccination, surgery, pregnancy, trauma, or stress, which activates the immune-mediated inflammatory response in these patients [6]. Vaccination is considered a rare trigger, with approximately 4.3% of antecedent events of NA [4,6]. NA also occurs as a hereditary disease, which is an autosomal dominant disorder with characteristic features such as earlier onset, higher recurrence rate, and worse long-term prognosis when compared with the idiopathic type. In 55% of the affected families, NA is associated with a point mutation or duplication in the SEPT9 gene on chromosome 17q25.3 [4,6,7]. In our case, the patient experienced her first shoulder drop following an HPV vaccination, and if NA recurs, genetic testing of the SEPT9 gene must be considered to discriminate hereditary NA.

HPV infection—caused by HPV types 16, 18, 31, and 45—is the major cause of cervical cancer [8]. HPV vaccination provides prophylaxis against HPV infection and related diseases, such as genital warts and cervical cancer [9]. Furthermore, even in previously HPV-infected women, HPV vaccination is important because it helps prevent the spread of infection to others [10]. This vaccination is advantageous in conferring protection against persistent HPV type 16 and 18 infections for 7 years. Moreover, HPV type 16 and 18 infections are more likely to be eliminated in vaccinated women than in unvaccinated women [11]. It appears to affect an earlier clearance of HPV infection in patients who have tested positive for HPV DNA [10].

The common adverse effects of an HPV vaccine are injection site discomfort—such as pain, swelling, and redness—due to an inflammatory response to virus-like particles [8,9]. It can also lead to systemic symptoms such as fever, nausea, vomiting, headache, dizziness, myalgia, and diarrhea [9]. Cases of autoimmune diseases following exposure to HPV vaccination are reported regularly, although there is no strong evidence that HPV vaccination increases the risk of autoimmune disease [12,13]. Thus, it would be necessary to verify more cases and constantly perform surveillance. In previous studies, only two cases of adverse effects presenting as NA after HPV vaccination have been reported to date, in which the patients presented with severe pain and paralysis in the region after the second HPV vaccination [14,15]. In our case, the patient complained of painless weakness in her shoulder after the first injection. We presumed that our patient presented with symptoms even after the first HPV vaccination because of the underlying HNPP. It might have been due to hereditary vulnerability to the occurrence of an immune-mediated NA.

Our patient only had a clinical presentation of NA after HPV vaccination; however, the electrodiagnostic findings led us to suspect underlying diffuse polyneuropathy. Inflammatory demyelinating polyneuropathy was excluded because of the negative results of cerebrospinal fluid analysis and brachial plexus MRI. Genetic testing demonstrated *PMP 22* deletion, which is the key feature of HNPP. The child did not meet the other criteria for HNPP diagnosis, which are as follows: autosomal dominant family history, age at symptom onset around the second decade, and rapid onset sensorimotor deficit preceded by a minor injury [1]. However, HNPP in pediatric patients has been reported as a phenotype of diffuse demyelinating polyneuropathy [2]. The parents of our patient declined the offer of genetic counselling; thus, we could not obtain information regarding family history of HNPP, which was a limitation of this case study.

In our patient, NA was potentially triggered by an immune-mediated inflammatory response due to HPV vaccination [5]. Remiche et al. reported that genetically determined neuropathy might affect immune-related peripheral neuropathy [16]. It has been suggested that hereditary neuropathy could predispose patients to the development of immune-mediated neuropathy [16]. In previous studies, cases of the associations between genetic and inflammatory neuropathies have been reported; thus, it might be necessary to consider genetic disorders in the process of diagnosing neuropathy [17]. The patient's concomitant HNPP vulnerability to pressure may be severely worsened due to virus-like particle-related immune reactions against the brachial plexus near the vaccination site.

To the best of our knowledge, this is the first case reporting the comorbidity of NA after HPV vaccination and underlying HNPP. HPV vaccination may potentially cause NA in patients with pre-existing HNPP due to an immune reaction. The asymptomatic HNPP might be vulnerable to the occurrence of an NA as the cause of a dropped shoulder. Our case report demonstrates a possible association between the NA and HNPP. The observation of potential factors that might suggest HNPP in patients with NA by comparing the differences between the reported cases will be of great importance and worth examining in future studies. This study highlights the importance of assessing clinical, electrodiagnostic, and genetic findings to make an accurate diagnosis of NA after HPV vaccination in a patient with pre-existing HNPP. Clinicians should consider hereditary neuropathy as a possible predisposing disease for the development of immune-mediated neuropathy. There may be genetic and immunological associations between HNPP and NA, which require further investigation.

Author Contributions: Conceptualization, H.-C.A. and J.-H.C.; methodology, J.-H.C.; software, D.-H.K.; validation, C.-H.C., J.-C.B. and D.-H.K.; formal analysis, H.-C.A.; investigation, H.-C.A.; resources, J.-C.B.; data curation, D.-H.K.; writing—original draft preparation, H.-C.A.; writing—review and editing, J.-H.C.; visualization, D.-H.K.; supervision, D.-H.K.; project administration, J.-H.C.; funding acquisition, J.-H.C. All authors have read and agreed to the published version of the manuscript.

Funding: This research was supported by the Bisa Research Grant of Keimyung University in 2020.

Institutional Review Board Statement: The study was conducted according to the guidelines of the Declaration of Helsinki and approved by the Institutional Review Board of Keimyung University Dongsan Hospital (DSMC 2021-01-079).

Informed Consent Statement: Informed consent was obtained from the patient's legal guardian. Given the patient's age, assent was not required.

Data Availability Statement: Not applicable.

Conflicts of Interest: The authors declare no conflict of interest.

References

1. Attarian, S.; Fatehi, F.; Rajabally, Y.A.; Pareyson, D. Hereditary neuropathy with liability to pressure palsies. *J. Neurol.* **2020**, *267*, 2198–2206. [CrossRef] [PubMed]
2. Chrestian, N.; McMillan, H.; Poulin, C.; Campbell, C.; Vajsar, J. Hereditary neuropathy with liability to pressure palsies in childhood: Case series and literature update. *Neuromuscul. Disord.* **2015**, *25*, 693–698. [CrossRef] [PubMed]
3. Van Eijk, J.J.; Groothuis, J.T.; Van Alfen, N. Neuralgic amyotrophy: An update on diagnosis, pathophysiology, and treatment. *Muscle Nerve* **2016**, *53*, 337–350. [CrossRef] [PubMed]
4. Kim, T.U.; Chang, M.C. Neuralgic amyotrophy: An underrecognized entity. *J. Int. Med. Res.* **2021**, *49*, 3000605211006542. [CrossRef] [PubMed]
5. Kim, S.I.; Seok, H.Y.; Yi, J.; Cho, J.H. Leg paralysis after AstraZeneca COVID-19 vaccination diagnosed as neuralgic amyotrophy of the lumbosacral plexus: A case report. *J. Int. Med. Res.* **2021**, *49*, 3000605211056783. [CrossRef] [PubMed]
6. Van Alfen, N.; van Engelen, B.G. The clinical spectrum of neuralgic amyotrophy in 246 cases. *Brain* **2006**, *129*, 438–450. [CrossRef] [PubMed]
7. Van Alfen, N. Clinical and pathophysiological concepts of neuralgic amyotrophy. *Nat. Rev. Neurol.* **2011**, *7*, 315–322. [CrossRef] [PubMed]
8. Huang, R.; Gan, R.; Zhang, D.; Xiao, J. The comparative safety of human papillomavirus vaccines: A Bayesian network meta-analysis. *J. Med. Virol.* **2022**, *94*, 729–736. [CrossRef] [PubMed]
9. Cheng, L.; Wang, Y.; Du, J. Human Papillomavirus Vaccines: An Updated Review. *Vaccines* **2020**, *8*, 391. [CrossRef] [PubMed]
10. Valasoulis, G.; Pouliakis, A.; Michail, G.; Kottaridi, C.; Spathis, A.; Kyrgiou, M.; Paraskevaidis, E.; Daponte, A. Alterations of HPV-Related Biomarkers after Prophylactic HPV Vaccination. A Prospective Pilot Observational Study in Greek Women. *Cancers* **2020**, *12*, 1164. [CrossRef] [PubMed]
11. Sasieni, P. Alternative analysis of the data from a HPV vaccine study in India. *Lancet Oncol.* **2022**, *23*, E9. [CrossRef]
12. Gidengil, C.; Goetz, M.B.; Newberry, S.; Maglione, M.; Hall, O.; Larkin, J.; Motala, A.; Hempel, S. Safety of vaccines used for routine immunization in the United States: An updated systematic review and meta-analysis. *Vaccine* **2021**, *39*, 3696–3716. [CrossRef] [PubMed]
13. Grimaldi-Bensouda, L.; Rossignol, M.; Kone-Paut, I.; Krivitzky, A.; Lebrun-Frenay, C.; Clet, J.; Brassat, D.; Papeix, C.; Nicolino, M.; Benhamou, P.Y.; et al. Risk of autoimmune diseases and human papilloma virus (HPV) vaccines: Six years of case-referent surveillance. *J. Autoimmun.* **2017**, *79*, 84–90. [CrossRef] [PubMed]
14. Debeer, P.; De Munter, P.; Bruyninckx, F.; Devlieger, R. Brachial plexus neuritis following HPV vaccination. *Vaccine* **2008**, *26*, 4417–4419. [CrossRef] [PubMed]
15. Taras, J.S.; King, J.J.; Jacoby, S.M.; McCabe, L.A. Brachial neuritis following quadrivalent human papilloma virus (HPV) vaccination. *Hand* **2011**, *6*, 454–456. [CrossRef] [PubMed]
16. Remiche, G.; Abramowicz, M.; Mavroudakis, N. Chronic inflammatory demyelinating polyradiculoneuropathy (CIDP) associated to hereditary neuropathy with liability to pressure palsies (HNPP) and revealed after influenza AH1N1 vaccination. *Acta Neurol. Belg.* **2013**, *113*, 519–522. [CrossRef] [PubMed]
17. Rajabally, Y.A.; Adams, D.; Latour, P.; Attarian, S. Hereditary and inflammatory neuropathies: A review of reported associations, mimics and misdiagnoses. *J. Neurol. Neurosurg. Psychiatry* **2016**, *87*, 1051–1060. [CrossRef] [PubMed]

MDPI
St. Alban-Anlage 66
4052 Basel
Switzerland
Tel. +41 61 683 77 34
Fax +41 61 302 89 18
www.mdpi.com

Children Editorial Office
E-mail: children@mdpi.com
www.mdpi.com/journal/children

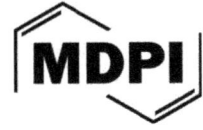

www.ingramcontent.com/pod-product-compliance
Lightning Source LLC
LaVergne TN
LVHW070607100526
838202LV00012B/585